Don't Squeeze the Spaceman's Taco

Lessons Learned from My Son

with Autism

by

Kelly Jude Melerine

Don't Squeeze the Spaceman's Taco

This is a story about autism and what a family does to stay strong.

Copyright © 2018 by Kelly Jude Melerine

Cover photo by Lauren Adelle Woods

Chapter 1

Sometime the Mighty Oak Falls

Cade Brent Melerine was born on a steamy summer afternoon in New Orleans, Louisiana. Little did I realize just how much my life was going to change. I'd taken care of many nieces, nephews and godchildren, but Cade would be the first of my own. My first born son. The first of five; that was my initial plan. You see, I was a natural at making children laugh. After all, that's what uncles and godfathers do. We make them laugh; we have a good time; we feed them junk food and we send them home.

But Cade would be the first that we couldn't send home. There he was, still covered in a mass of white greasy goo. He looked like something out of a science fiction horror movie. Actually, he was rather adorable once the nurse cleaned him up. His infant-sized lungs filled with air as he cried for the very first time.

I remember holding that beautiful slime covered baby tightly, hoping not to drop him. Slowly I swayed until his crying stopped. His dark colored eyes opened wide as he took in this new world around him.

"So Helena's a boy." Julee smiled as I laid Cade upon her chest.

We didn't want to know the sex of the baby beforehand. We wanted it to be a surprise. And surprised we were. I had just painted the baby room a soft pastel yellow. We figured it was a nice neutral color. I also painted an image of Tinkerbell fluttering about the bassinet while leaving a trail of pixie dust in her midst. Ok, so we had a strong feeling that we were having a girl. Helena Janice Melerine would be named after both of her grandmothers. But instead, Cade was named after his place of conception.

Cade's Cove is a charming valley nestled within the Great Smoky Mountains of Tennessee. A week-long getaway brought home a lifetime of memories.

My name is Kelly Jude Melerine and I'm a stay at home dad of a teenage boy with autism named Cade. I quit my job in banking following an extremely rough phase with him. Since then I've become a jack of all trades just to pay the bills. I juggle many tasks so that I may keep a flexible schedule and continue my daily focus on my son. My wife Julee maintains her job as an office manager. Her job provides additional income for the family as well as medical benefits. My son has made tremendous progress with me at home but it's a constant struggle. However, it's a struggle that I will gladly face for him each day.

    This isn't a typical self-help guide to coping with autism and nor should it be treated as such. Life with autism is anything but typical. This is a story of family. Not the type that you see on TV commercials with perfectly decorated homes and saintly well-behaved children. But the type of family that breaks the rules, kicks holes in walls and makes spectacles in public places. This is a story of life. Not the type that most would strive to achieve. But the type of life that tests your limits, beats you down and leaves you in a constant state of turmoil. It's is a story of lessons learned through heartache and chaos. It's about taking a shit sandwich and turning it into a fully dressed shrimp po-boy. It's about laughter through tears and strength through forgiveness. It's about facing unthinkable challenges and tackling our biggest fears no matter how ill prepared we are.

The greatest of all these challenges occurred in the summer of 2011. Cade was admitted to the hospital twice for what his doctors referred to as psychotic behavior. During his second hospital stay we were faced with the recommendation of having him institutionalized. His early teenage years were plagued with episodes of extreme violence. As Cade became bigger and stronger, so did his violent outbursts. The attacks, however were only directed towards my wife Julee and me. He somehow managed to keep it together for everyone else. What his doctors viewed as a solution I viewed as a nightmare. Convinced that a parent can make a difference, I took matters into my own hands.

You see, Cade had been on various medications for most of his life. Contrary to doctor's orders I believed that the medication was the root of my son's violence. Rather than send him to a long term facility we decided to take him home and wean him off all of his crazy meds. His behavior improved almost immediately. No longer were Cade's violent attacks directed towards Julee. He would still, however sock it to me at times. It was during these times that I believed that he was in pain. My gut feeling told me that Cade was suffering from migraines or other severe headaches. Convincing doctors that a special needs child is in pain requires persistence. Unfortunately, when it comes to children with disabilities, doctors are quick to label everything as behavioral problems.

A breakthrough in my son's pain relief came two years later while vacationing in central Florida. Cade loves roller coasters and other amusement park thrill rides. Orlando is the perfect place for him to fulfill his thrill seeking desires. Traveling with autism requires planning and theme parks are only visited during their slower seasons. The key thing being shorter wait times. Cheaper hotel rates are just a bonus. Besides, Cade doesn't mind missing a few days of school if it means having a little fun.

Universal Studios, home of Cade's favorite ride – *The Mummy*. It's September 2013, a week after Labor Day and two years since his last hospital stay. We approach the turnstile to the attraction when I notice there's something wrong.

"When you going to Uncle Darrin's house?" Cade asks with a glazed look in his eyes.

For some reason he asks this question when he is experiencing pain. Cade also speaks of himself in the third person. Everyone else says "you" when referring to him. Therefore, Cade does the same. Being the parent of a child with limited verbal skills, you quickly learn their unique nuances. Vibrations are felt as the train enters the station to board new passengers. Anxiously, the crowd stands by awaiting the two minutes of excitement promised by this attraction. Who knew that we would be the ones providing the excitement? And then it starts. Fiercely and with the precision of a rapid fire assault rifle, Cade spits vigorously upon my face. Struggling to remain calm, I do my best to discretely exit. Before long my shirt is ripped to shreds and Cade bites down like a savage dog. This is what we call being discrete.

Moments later the park's medics arrive. Julee removes a bottle of Excedrine from her purse and we ask for a Coke. I explain that caffeine usually helps and that we just need some quiet time. Observing Cade in his current state, anti-psychotic drugs are recommended for sedation. I refuse. Guarding my child, we argue back and forth until the ambulance arrives.

"This isn't what a headache looks like," the medic insists.

"This isn't what a headache looks like to a typical person," I agree. "But you are talking about someone that can't verbalize, 'My fucking head is killing me.'"

Cade is wheeled into the ambulance upon a gurney. Sweat drips down my back from the heat of the scuffle and the Florida sun. Leaning forward, I peal myself from the front seat. Cade still desperately wants to kick my ass so it's not safe for me to ride in the back. Through the glass opening, I painfully watch as my son cries. Undoubtedly, he hates being strapped down. With what remains of my smiley face t-shirt I wrap my forearm tightly. Julee and her brother Brett head back to the hotel room. Julee's brother lives with us as well. Brett is a grown man in his forties. However, due to brain damage, he remains eternally twelve. I send Julee a text message as we approach the local hospital.

"Everything is going well."

"What do you want scuba squat?" Right away I know that Brett has Julee's phone.

"Tell Julee that Cade is calm and not to worry." Of course, this is a lie and Cade continues screaming in the back. I take one last deep breath as the vehicle pulls up to the emergency room entrance.

The glass doors part and we enter the hospital. I maintain a comfortable distance to keep from upsetting Cade. It's the typical emergency room atmosphere. People are shuffling about rapidly. The smell of Lysol fills the air. Code phrases echo from the PA system alerting the medical staff. I don't know their code for "Out of control kid with stubborn parent." But I'm pretty sure I heard it.

The medic from the park gives his assessment and then I give mine.

"The sooner he gets treatment for his headache, the sooner he will quiet down." This I urge the doctor. I inform her that Cade has a history of severe headaches and migraines. "I know that this doesn't look like a typical headache patient," I continue. "But Cade has autism and with his limited words this is how he expresses his pain."

Then, something unexpected happens. She listens. While his doctors back home drew their own conclusions, she actually listens. There I stand, shirtless and shivering. I'm shocked to have a medical professional actually listening to me.

A few minutes later, a kind elderly lady approaches and wraps me in a warm blanket. She has the most soothing voice. Her husband recently passed away and she's back at work escaping her newfound loneliness. Her encouraging words help to put my mind at ease. Before leaving, she hands me a hospital gown.

"I know it's not very stylish." She chuckles. "I mean, who designs these things anyway? Probably some *Project Runway* reject." Before leaving the room, she pats my hand. "If you need anything, I'll be around. I'm going to call Heidi Klum and tell her what I think about these awful gowns."

Intravenously, the nurse administers medication for Cade's headache pain. Shortly after an injection of Imitrex, Cade becomes calm and relaxed.

"I'm sorry Dad," he sobs. "I tore your shirt."

"Yeah buddy." I can't help but laugh. "You tore my shirt."

But I also want to cry. Cade said two complete sentences. Hearing those words was pure magic. It was like being back at the amusement park marveling over the latest attraction their engineers dreamed up.

The medic from the park approaches and taps me on the shoulder.

"I must apologize. This is a big lesson learned for me. You're one heck of a father," he continues. "Please accept my apology."

"Apology accepted."

With matching gowns we exit the hospital. The rest of the day is spent relaxing quietly in our hotel room.

Two days later we take home more than just the usual tacky souvenirs. We take home proof that Cade is experiencing pain. Without hesitation, I drop Cade's neurologist and schedule an appointment with our family doctor. We give him the records from the Florida hospital. With confidence, he writes a prescription for Imitrex to be taken as needed. I can't tell you how many times that prescription has saved the day.

It was when I tucked Cade in that night that it hit me. There he is, lying in bed. His assortment of furry stuffed animals is gathered around him like he's part of the herd. Cade's smile is even bigger than the one on Manny. Manny is by far Cade's favorite bear. The thought of my son locked up in a facility freaked out on crazy meds goes ravaging through my mind. The idea of him being in pain on top of all this becomes overwhelming.

Repeatedly, the words of the park's medic echo in my head. "You're one heck of a father." Uncontrollably, I start to cry. A tear falls upon Cade's Superman quilt and I wipe it off. Masking my sorrow, I smile and wish Cade a good night.

As I click off his light switch I hear Julee calling my name.

"Did you feed the dogs?"

Thinking to myself, it was clear. I forgot to buy dog food. "Shit!"

Tramp and Gumbo gather around as if reading my mind. Wagging their tails they lead me to the back door.

"I'll be right back," I shout. "I need to pick up a couple items from the grocery store."

"Did you forget to buy dog food today?" She asks from the bathroom.

"No, of course not." Julee always knows when I'm lying. "Do you need me to get anything while I am there?"

"We could use more coffee."

"Cool. I'll be right back."

Walking pass the bathroom window a familiar smile peeks through the blinds. Tapping on the glass, Julee snickers. "They like Kibbles 'n Bits."

It's a little past ten o'clock and the local Bi-Lo is already closed. I really hate roaming through Walmart for just a few items but Tramp and Gumbo gave me orders. Aimlessly, I walk the aisles that night. "Dog food and coffee." I remind myself. "Dog food and coffee." I must have made that loop five or six times before stopping. "Kibbles 'n Bits." With both hands I lift the bag and continue roaming. Repeatedly, I beat myself up over how long Cade has been suffering with headaches. There's no escaping the thought of him being institutionalized and tormented the rest of his life. The words of the medic play over and over, "You're one heck of a father." Knowing how long Cade has been in pain made me doubt those words even more. A few extra passes down the coffee aisle and my trip to Walmart is complete. Avoiding human contact, I scan my items at the self-checkout lane and leave the building. Leaning over the driver's side window, a dreaded image appears.

"Shit!" I bang my head against the car's window. "That's just great."

With my keys locked inside the vehicle, I give Julee a call. A familiar voice picks up on the other end but it's certainly not my wife. It's Shakira. Uncontrollably, my toes start tapping to the beat of "My Hips Don't Lie." I shake my head as I picture Julee soaking care free in the tub with her phone vibrating somewhere deep within the pockets of her red leather purse.

Immediately, I press redial. The catchy Latin hook of her callback ringtone lets me know one thing. It's time to start walking.

"No big deal." I tell myself. "It's just a couple miles." With a pound of coffee and thirty-five pounds of dog food I start my journey.

I get about half way home before stopping on the tracks of an abandoned railroad crossing. Conveniently, the hefty bag of Kibbles 'n Bits makes for a comfy bean bag like seat. Slowly, my body shifts as I think about my son. The tension in my neck quickly escalates. In small circles, I rotate my head; just enough to ease the stress a bit. And that's when I feel it. I've been wearing my mom's old St. Jude medal. Observing it under the light of the street post I begin to smile. "The patron saint of lost causes," I think to myself. "What do I have to lose?" We sit there a few minutes, St. Jude and I. One solution keeps coming to mind. Quit my job and stay home with Cade. Not permanently, but long enough to get him through this current state of madness. Gently, I pull the medal towards my lips and softly give it a kiss. My fingers glide across the etched surface as I tuck it back under my shirt. Closing my eyes, I relive the day that I received Mom's medal. Admittedly, I was never the best Catholic. But thank you St. Jude and thank you Mom.

My mother was always a very religious woman. More importantly, she had faith. I've never known anyone more kind, generous and pure of heart. The crazy thing is that she didn't always see herself that way. Her deep devotion to the Catholic religion caused her to view herself as a sinner. Strangely enough, she never viewed anyone else in that manner. The critical views she had of herself led her to multiple nervous breakdowns. I remember my first time visiting her at the state mental hospital.

I was twelve-years-old back then. The trek across the Causeway Bridge seemed like an eternity. The bridge crossed Lake Pontchartrain just north of New Orleans. Stretching over twenty-four miles, Guinness World Records lists the Causeway Bridge as the longest bridge over water in the world. And long it was. Especially to a kid eager to see his mother. The warm humid air brushed through my wavy brown hair as I stuck my head out of the window.

"Get your head back in the car," my sister yelled from the driver's seat.

Iris was my biggest role model growing up. She was fifteen years older than me. In many ways she was my sister, mother and friend. My parents had three children a little over a year apart. Then fourteen years later there were two more. That's where I came in. I was their final accident. Lucky for me, the rhythm method was about the only form of birth control approved by the Catholic Church.

I stared at the endless horizon of water. The only thing I had to occupy my time was that stupid punch buggy game. For the past eighteen miles there's been nothing but water; not a single punch buggy around. With not much else to do, I stuck my head back out of the window.

"You better listen to your sister!" Reaching through the passenger side window, my father slapped my head back into the car. That man really had a way with words.

Nestled among wooded acres in the small town of Mandeville was the state mental hospital. Although now a thriving community, Mandeville was once synonymous with psychiatric care. Anyone going to Mandeville was either crazy themselves or had crazy in the family. It just depended on which side of the door they were standing.

And there I stood, on the right side of sanity. I remember rocking back and forth with the movement of the tall pine trees. Carefully I observed the hospital door as I anxiously awaited my mom. I hadn't seen her in over two weeks and I was missing her terribly. I gazed back up towards the tall pines. I watched as they swayed continuously in the wind. There were many varieties of trees in those woods but I clearly remember the pines. I admired their constant fight to stand tall despite the opposing winds. I watched for a moment then shifted back to the door. Nervously I waited for the slightest movement. The smell of summer breezed through the air and I continued swaying. Back and forth I remained with the movement of the trees.

There were two things that I knew for certain. I really wanted to see my mother and I really needed to pee. Standing majestically among the landscape were centuries old oak trees. Quickly I darted behind one of the oaks. Scared that I'd miss the moment that Mom came through the door, I unzipped my pants. With my head leaning around the side of the tree's massive trunk, I let the waters flow. My eyes remained focused at the door. While zipping up my khaki shorts a streak of red caught my eye. I glanced upwards and it was a kite made by one of the patients. A strong gust carried it and away went the kite. Higher and higher, I watched as the kite continued to soar. The trees remained swaying. Their narrow forms stood reaching high with their limbs rocking to and fro. Skittishly, I shifted my eyes back to the door.

My body remained swaying until the door finally opened. And there she was; just as beautiful as ever. The wind gently parted her thick dark hair. Her sapphire eyes sparkled as she glanced my way. Immediately, I ran and embraced her. The hour that I spent with her that day I will always cherish.

Contently I sat as Mom, Dad and my sister engaged in conversation. Honestly, I was happy just sitting there. My eyes scanned the park like setting. Observing the other families I couldn't help but wonder, "What brought them here?" Even at that young of an age I remember being worried. "Could I end up here?" I thought of the many storms that have passed through those woods. Although many trees still stood tall, many have given way to the pressures of life and snapped. There's a breaking point when even the mightiest oak tree falls.

Minutes later a middle-aged man riding on a horse galloped towards us. With reference to me, he greeted my sister. "Ma'am, I just saved your little boy." Graciously, he accepted my sister's thanks and then rode off into the crowd. The horse, by the way, was only in his mind.

"Where was he going?" I wondered. Apparently it was somewhere in a world that he created himself. Many of the patients here lived in their own universe. They seemed happy enough though.

And then there was that part of the hospital where children weren't allowed to visit. Mom made reference to the terrible noises that came from there. I envisioned a fortress covered in a cloud of darkness. Was this dark world a place that they created themselves? Or maybe, this darkness was their reality? And unlike the other happy patients here, they just haven't been able to create a perfect utopia for them to escape. The real world can be overwhelming and even menacing at times. Escaping doesn't necessarily mean that you're crazy. It's how you've escaped that determines this.

Saying good-bye was really hard that day. However, Mom assured me that she was going to be all right. She believed that she was sent here to find healing. Tightly I hugged her as she handed me a note.

"The Physician"

The healing hands that He did give
To heal the lame and blind
The warming touch of His embrace
There's strength unto the mind
The ER doctor has his way
He prays to God above
Let me console the open wounds
And ease the pain with love
The psychiatric doctor cares
He's there to understand
Give wisdom to my knowledge Lord
He reaches to your hand
The surgeon does your work Dear Lord
His skills are learned with care
Consoling with your help each day
There's healing everywhere
The doctor of your church my Lord
He came to heal the soul
The peace and joy that come within
The greatest story told

Helen Melerine

I spotted eight punch buggies on the way home. It's funny how the ride back didn't seem so long. My bladder however, was filled to capacity and I needed relief. Pulling up my shirt to reach my pants, I felt a sudden sting. There was a tic attached to my naval and it was burrowing deeper into my skin. With a swift jerk I managed to pull it out. "There," I thought to myself, "that wasn't so bad." A few seconds later and I'm running out of the bathroom with my pants around my knees screaming horrifically.

"Get it off…Get it off!" I yelled.

"What's wrong?" asked Iris.

"There's a tic on my wiener!" I shouted. "I tried pulling it off but it just dug deeper."

"What?" she asked in disbelief.

"There's a tic on my wiener!" again I shouted.

My father immediately burst into laughter. And then, the unimaginable happened.

"Let me see." My sister pulled tweezers from her purse.

"You don't need tweezers!" I frantically yelled. "My wiener's not that small."

Trying her best not to laugh, she insisted, "It's for the tic. Now let me take a look at that thing."

There I stood with my withered schnitzel in front of my sister. Believe me, it was the last thing I wanted to do at the kitchen table. But this was an emergency and it couldn't possibly get any worse.

Just then, my brother Darrin walked into the kitchen with a group of his friends. Before long, the story of the kid with a tic on his dick spread throughout the entire neighborhood. And that's when I learned the hazards of peeing in the woods.

With the tic gone I let out a sigh of relief. My sister's next three words; however, made me cringe.

"Need some alcohol."

It wasn't all together bad when I got home though. My father handed me my mother's St. Jude medal and said that she wanted me to have it. I've been wearing it ever since.

Drifting back to reality, I slowly rise from my smashed sack of Kibbles 'n Bits. I lift the bag over my shoulder and continue walking home. "We have one year to get this right," I tell myself. That's about all the time the funds I have saved for retirement will allow. Our nest egg had been depleted several times in the past. The first time was during Cade's early years. Bills from doctors and therapists were through the roof. Intensive speech and occupational therapies were showing positive signs in the treatment of autism. Unfortunately, insurance coverage for these types of treatments was usually limited to stroke patients and accident victims. Retirement funds drained. The second blow to our retirement came in 2005 when Hurricane Katrina wiped out everything else that we owned in southern Louisiana. Retirement funds drained again. Eight years later, I have a sack of dog food on my shoulder and budget cuts on my mind. Quitting my job is a big risk. Quitting my son is a bigger risk. Good bye retirement.

The soothing sound of a jazz saxophone echoes as I pass the bathroom window. I enter the house and Tramp and Gumbo guide me directly to their bowls.

"A little kibble for you." Immediately Tramp dives in.

"And some bits for you." Gumbo follows shortly behind.

I take a couple wine glasses back to Julee. The lavender candles and soft tunes were a nice touch to our otherwise outdated powder blue bathroom. Extending my finger, I shush her as she attempts to speak. Silently I sit on the edge of the tub. Julee leans back and we let the saxophone do the talking. After so many years together, there's often no need for words. We usually know what the other one is thinking.

"Do you believe the price of coffee went up almost a dollar?" I sigh.

"OK?" She mutters questionably, giving me that obvious eye roll. "Why don't you join me in the bubbles?"

Fully dressed, I lean back into the tub. We spend the next several minutes laughing about all the crap that we've been through.

"Wait a minute." I tell her. "I've got just the right thing."

Water cascades down my pants as I step out of the tub. I scan Julee's IPod and make my final selection. Dripping wet, I lip sync into the toilet plunger. "Promise Me You'll Remember" by Harry Connick Jr was the song I dedicated to her on our wedding day in 1992.

It takes quite a few bath towels to dry the floor that evening. While cleaning on our hands and knees, Julee looks towards me.

"Maybe I should take a leave of absence," reluctantly she suggests.

"Really?"

"Yeah," she replies, "the guys that I work with are very understanding."

"Well," I pause and then continue. "I was actually thinking that I should be the one staying home. I know that he hasn't gotten violent with you in a long time but he is a big boy."

"I really don't believe that he would hurt me anymore," she asserts. "But you're right. He is a big boy."

"Much bigger than you. Besides, the only time that he has an outburst now is when he has a headache. I can just give him his pill and then hide somewhere in the house. He's terrible at hide and seek." I chuckle a bit and continue. "If I hide then I won't have to wrestle him."

"How long were you thinking?" She asks.

I sit back along the edge of the tub. "About a year. We should be able to stretch things a year. I can get a part time job if I have to."

Tears stream from Julee's eyes. "I think that Cade really needs this right now…Oh no!" Sniffling, she adds, "What about Nellie?"

I'm a bank manager and Nellie is my assistant. She's also one of the best souls that I've ever met. "I'll give them all the time that they need to find a replacement. I won't leave Nellie with just anybody."

Julee comes in for a hug. I fall back and into the tub we go for the second time. Coming up from the bubbles, Julee rests her sudsy red hair against my chest.

"Thank you," she whispers.

"You are very welcome. Plus think of all the delicious meals that I can prepare."

"Maybe this is a dumb idea after all," she laughs.

We recall my many failed attempts at dinner. Soon after we were married it was resolved that Julee would be in charge of the cooking and I would take care of the cleaning. This resolution came after my catastrophic experiment with spaghetti and meatballs. It was a mid-week evening and Julee was working late. A romantic candle lit dinner sounded like a nice surprise.

"No need for a recipe," I thought to myself.

I've seen the chefs on television. It's just a pinch of this and a pinch of that.

"I can do this."

A dozen pinches later and still there was something missing.

"What would Emeril do?" I asked myself.

And that's when I decided to add a little wine. Truthfully, I'm no sommelier. Therefore, the cheap bottle of Asti Spumante from the Dirty Santa gift exchange seemed like a good idea. Slowly, I added the sparkling white wine to the canned sauce and stirred. Not wanting to be wasteful, I poured the rest of that cheap shit into my meatball mixture.

The table was set and Julee and I had our seats. Quietly we stared at the pink mush. Twirling her fork, Julee courageously took the first bite while I continued staring at this repulsive mound of pink rubbish.

"You know," I told her. "I've really been wanting to try that new seafood restaurant."

Needless to say, she agreed and that was the best catfish dinner ever.

Chapter 2

Prescription for Disaster

I'm sure that most people have heard the phrase, "I feel your pain." It's merely a way of showing empathy. But, have you ever become so in tune with a person that you really do feel their pain? During the first years of life children count on their parents to notice any signs of discomfort or ailment. Since day one I have been attentively observing Cade. Continuously I watch for the slightest clues. When he laughs I laugh and when he hurts I hurt. It's a bond that's hard to describe.

Therapies and treatments for autism have wiped out our savings and maxed out our credit cards. From natural alternatives to strong pharmaceuticals, we've tried them all. I will never forget the look on Cade's face at his fourth birthday party. Cade was on the Feingold diet, sometime referred to as the ADHD diet. Through a process of elimination, foods containing certain additives are removed and then replaced by foods that are free of these additives. It was worth a shot.

<u>Here's what happened on the Feingold diet:</u>

The children gathered around Cade singing "Happy Birthday." They just spent the past two hours destroying an inflatable bounce house and they were ready for some cake. Through a process of elimination, Cade's chocolate cupcake with chocolate icing was replaced by a buckwheat cupcake with carob icing. Although, no improvement was noted on the diet, the only side effect was wasted cupcakes.

Here's what happened next:

Not achieving the desired results, we turned to the medical professionals. Wasted cupcakes were soon replaced by rapid weight gain, anxiety, dry mouth, excessive perspiration, inability to perspire, warm sensations, hot sensations, sleepiness, sleeplessness, constipation, diarrhea, dizziness, muscle pain, joint pain and migraines – just to name a few. And to make matters worse, Cade can't explain these feelings.

This is when shit gets real. It was the summer of 2010 -- nine years since Cade's last buckwheat cupcake. He had just returned home from his favorite place in the world, Camp Sunshine. Camp Sunshine is a week-long celebration for individuals with disabilities. The event takes place in the sweltering heat of southern Mississippi. Cade looks forward to camp all year. His birthday usually falls during camp so we celebrate when he gets home.

Cade was thirteen years old at the time and on a once daily dosage of Abilify. The two of us sat down for an important discussion.

"So tell me Cade." I asked, "What type of cake would you like for your birthday?"

"Um, let's see," he pondered. "How about a Batman cake?"

"A Batman cake sounds awesome!" I exclaimed. Of course, this wouldn't be his first Batman cake. "What type of cake though?"

"A Batman cake," he repeated.

"Do you want a chocolate Batman cake?"

"Chocolate Batman cake!" With the enthusiasm of a varsity cheerleader, Cade made his final selection.

"Okay. A chocolate Batman cake it is."

While seated at the dining room table, Cade compiled a list of all the things that he wanted for his birthday. In bright orange crayon, the word Batman appeared at least a dozen times. Suddenly, he froze. Not because he ran out of Caped Crusader novelty items, mind you. But because he just froze. Uncontrollably, Cade's eyes rolled back and his muscles began to stiffen. Loud and with the pitch of a turbine engine, he screamed. Startled, I ran towards my son.

"What's wro…" Before I could ask, Cade was back to his list.

Several more items appeared on his list. And several more Batman's also appeared. Suddenly he froze.

"Cade?" I asked for his attention. "Cade?...Cade?"

Dropping in agony, he began to bang his head. An overwhelming feeling of helplessness overcame me as I tried to comfort him. For forty minutes straight he continued to scream and for forty minutes straight he pounded his head. Praying for Cade's relief, I could feel the sting of my own temples pulsating and pounding.

With the determination of a desperate parent, I shook off my pessimism and started searching for answers. Among numerous forums I encountered other individuals complaining of migraine headaches while taking Abilify. Concerned, I consulted with Cade's doctor.

"Don't tell me," leaning back in his chair the doctor clicked his pen, "Web MD?"

"I realize that I'm no expert," bending closer I continued. "It's just that Cade can't tell me how these medications make him feel. I admit that I don't know the chemistry behind the way that these medicines work. But I do know that my son is hurting."

"I understand your concern Mr. Melerine." Laying down his pen, Cade's doctor assured me. "I'm here to help. While what you're witnessing may appear to look like physical pain, head banging is a psychotic behavior."

"No." I told him, "Cade's not psychotic. He's hurting. I can tell."

With convincing from the doctor, Julee and I agreed. We exchanged our worries for a prescription to Cade's well-being. After all, the right medication can work wonders and mental health care has come a long way since my mother's days in Mandeville. An antipsychotic drug could very well be the breakthrough that we'd been hoping for.

Zyprexa, Risperdal, Seroquel and Geodon turned Cade into Freddy Krueger, Michael Myers, Jason and Chucky. He became extremely violent and attacked at any moment. Driving even short distances with Cade suddenly became dangerous. New holes were smashed into the walls as quickly as I could patch them. Fortunately, growing up the son of a carpenter, I learned a few of my dad's trades along the way. I was continuously repairing doors, windows and furniture. Ashamed, I started fabricating stories to explain my many scratches, bite wounds and bruises. It was easier for me to say that I had a pet bear than to say that I was attacked by my child.

Cade's aggression continued to soar. Meals were left unattended on the stove while he hunted us down for ass whippings. I was forced to wrestle with my son for hours on end. No matter how long the battle, he just wouldn't get tired. That's when we discovered that he was lousy at hide and seek. Rather than duke it out, we simply hid in the tub. Our bathtub soon became our porcelain safe haven.

With each new medication, we discussed the increase in Cade's violent behaviors. The doctor always had one of two solutions. Either we increased the dosage of his current antipsychotic drug or we switched Cade to a different antipsychotic drug. The doctor was convinced that puberty was triggering my son's extreme violent mood swings. Doing as prescribed, Cade went through a series of medication changes. With each new change came a new antipsychotic drug. With each new change Cade's behavior grew progressively worse. With each new change I suggested that maybe the medication was the problem. With each new change my suggestion was dismissed. After all, why would a mind altering medication cause an individual to act any differently?

If it weren't for late night talks with my mom I don't think that I would have survived. Mom's words have always inspired and lifted me. Even as an adult, she has helped me to overcome the greatest of life's challenges. I kept a collection of the poems that she wrote in a drawer next to my bed. It became sort of a nightly ritual for me to reach out to her. Mom never did sleep very well. Maybe it was because she was a chronic worrier. Or maybe it was because she drank a full pot of coffee every day. Either way, I knew that I could call on her anytime that I needed her.

Mom was always a very kind and innocent woman; the complete opposite of my father. He was always a grumpy bastard. However, I loved that grumpy bastard nonetheless. My friends always compared my parents to Archie and Edith Bunker from TV's *All in the Family*. To be honest, it's a fairly accurate depiction.

It was a blue collared household. Dad was a carpenter -- at least until his first heart attack. Following his illness we scraped by on Social Security disability. To help supplement Dad's lost income, our summers were spent working on a shrimp boat. Dad steered the boat and my brother Darrin and I provided the labor. Our reward from my father: $10 per day. I always excelled at math and realized that if I worked seven days per week I could earn a potential $70. That may not sound like much. But to a kid with no money, $70 was indeed a lot of money. The other perk? In addition to what was sold on the docks, we caught enough with our trawl nets to eat shrimp nearly every single day. By the end of the season, our bills were paid and our freezer was full.

Mom was a homemaker. She rose early from bed every morning to prepare a hearty breakfast for the family. While I was off at school, Mom's day was spent cooking and cleaning. However, there was one break that she took on a daily basis. And that was at 11:00 am central; the local air time for *The Young and the Restless*. My mother never missed an episode. Anytime there was a break from school, I too would join her in this indulgence. Reluctantly, I got hooked. If there was a cliffhanger episode that occurred during spring break, I had no choice but to fake an illness so that I could stay home a couple days extra. Fortunately, Mom never caught on and I was able to stay in the know with what happened to Katherine Chancellor.

My mother was always home when I returned from school. This I knew I could count on. And there was always a hot cooked meal waiting for me. This too was a given. From shrimp creole to red beans and rice; Mom's kitchen was like perfume on the bayou. The neighbors always raved about her buttermilk-cornmeal fried chicken. But if you ask me, nothing beat her homemade yeast bread. Any time she baked a loaf, I stole a piece and stashed it in my bedroom closet. There was a brass framed three dimensional Jesus picture hanging on our living room wall.

It was hard walking past 3-D Jesus with my stolen bread, but I did it anyway. I just made up for it in confession.

To be truthful, I often lied during confession. I mentioned previously that I wasn't a good Catholic. And this is my confession now, so please forgive me.

Mom, on the other hand, could never tell a lie. For if she did, she would be damned for all eternity. At least that's how she saw it. Even as she beat herself down, Mom lifted everyone else up. To date, she remains my biggest source of inspiration.

Inspiration was something desperately needed while Cade was on the crazy meds. During these trying times, it wasn't uncommon for me to go to bed and to wake to Mom's words of encouragement. I was over forty and morning reading required a little extra time for my eyes to adjust.

> ...I needn't ask him for his grace
> It's always here with me
> He watches over me with care
> Forever he will be...
>
> *Helen Melerine*

"Thank you mom," I whispered to myself. Feeling optimistic, I laid my phone down on the nightstand.

There were some mornings that I imagined waking up to a typical kid or that Cade somehow outgrew his autism. I longed for an in-depth conversation with my son. I wanted to know everything he's been thinking all of these years. Have I been a good father? Or have I just been getting things wrong all this time? Rolling out of bed, I made my way to his room.

"Good morning buddy."

"Good morning Dad," He paused and then continued. "Breakfast."

"What would you like for breakfast?"

"McDonald's Daddy."

He wanted to get out. That was a good sign. "McDonald's it is."

Walking to the bedroom to get my keys I caught a glimpse of Cade in the bathroom mirror. He had just finished brushing his teeth and was now working on his hair. When it comes to hair product, he never really grasped the idea that less is more. The end result? A glob of sticky goo piled randomly around his head. It takes everything in me not to smooth it all out. But he's a teenager now and he wants to do it himself. Spiky on one side and smashed on the other, we headed out to McDonald's.

"Daddy who's that?"

"Who?" I asked for clarity.

"Who's that?" Again he questioned.

"Who's what?"

"Radio Dad. Who's that?"

Not sure who the artist was on the radio, I replied, "I don't know buddy."

"Who's that Dad?" He continued asking.

When Cade has a question he will not give up until he receives an answer. And "I don't know" is never an acceptable answer. Pulling to the side of the road, I Googled songs about alien sex and pockets on Shrek.

"That's Katy Perry and Kanye West." I informed him and resumed our drive to McDonald's.

"Daddy"

"Yes Cade?"

"What city is Katy Perry from? What city?"

The next several minutes were spent researching Katy Perry and all her various band members. Satisfied with his new found knowledge we continued our quest for breakfast. Shortly into resuming our drive, I could sense the storm that was brewing within.

"Why don't we get drive through and eat at home?" I asked.

Cade agreed and we placed our order. My body tensed as I prepared for the inevitable. Praying for a safe drive home, I reached for our items from the drive through window.

"Here are your coffees and your biscuits. If you don't mind…," I dreaded her coming words. "Would you pull up to the yellow line and wait for your breakfast burrito?"

Reluctantly, I did as instructed. That damn burrito was the only reason that we were there. Knowing that our time was limited, I called my cousin Pat. She lived close by and could take Cade home. Cade would never hurt Pat nor anyone else for that matter. No one other than Julee and me, that is. And driving home would just be too dangerous now.

Through the side mirror I watched the clerk approach. Delightfully, a smile stretched across her face. She was a pleasant young lady, undoubtedly happy with her new job. Meanwhile, inside the vehicle Cade was seated on the verge of a violent outburst. I watched as he suddenly ripped through the brown paper bag. In just one bite an entire biscuit was devoured. At that moment, the clerk gleefully tapped on my window. Lowering my window to reach for Cade's coveted burrito, I was abruptly jolted with pain.

"Fuck!" Uncontrollably, I screamed. Cade's teeth gripped down upon my shoulder.

"So sorry," I gave my apologies to the clerk.

"Is everything all right?"

"We're fine," I insisted as Cade spit biscuit crumbs across my windshield. I really hated to make a scene. More importantly, I hated having the police called. We'd been through that several times already and I just didn't want my son to be labeled as violent.

Cade started rambling in a crazed, maniacal manner. Leaping over the bag between us, he bit down again and again. My arm was pulverized. Hair putty oozed through my fingers as I pulled his head from my forearm.

"Cousin Pat will be here soon," I assured him. "Eat your burrito."

With closed fists Cade pounded the bag and his precious burrito bit the dust. He lunged towards me clamping his teeth onto my forearm. My coffee cup was crushed sending hot liquid pouring down my shirt. Worried that he may have gotten burned I pulled away and opened the door. Although there was a lot of screaming going on, there really was no telling if he was hurt. The only thing that was clear was that Cade wanted to inflict pain upon me and he wasn't going to stop anytime soon. Standing outside the vehicle with burrito guts hanging from my ear, again I tried to calm him down.

"Cousin Pat is almost here." I reassured. "We'll be going home soon."

"Going home soon!" Repeatedly, he shouted. "Going home soon! Going home soon! Going home soon!..."

Restlessly, he exited the passenger side door prompting me to retreat back in. Still somehow hoping to avoid making a spectacle, I locked all doors. Paralyzed in emotion, I sat there as Cade pelted the window. His face was blurred from the spit covering the glass. Determined that he was going to get to me, he started kicking in the door.

"Stop it Cade!" I shouted.

Again he kicked the door.

"You know what?" I yelled to myself. "Fuck this shit!"

Jumping out of the vehicle, I wrestled him to the ground. Blood dripped down my arm from my open wounds as I held Cade firmly in a head lock. We totally obliterated the shrubbery surrounding the golden arches that morning.

Thank God for family. Pat finally arrived and Cade willingly left with her. Police sirens passed as I followed shortly behind.

These violent outburst became all too familiar. Keeping my sanity was about as difficult as keeping my cool. Cade pushed my discipline to the limits.

Watching television while he repeatedly spit on my face...

"I'm stronger than this," I reminded myself.

Dining in a restaurant while he choked me with my necktie...

"I'm stronger than this."

Wrestling across restaurant tables while covered in spaghetti sauce, breadcrumbs and blood…

"I'm stronger than this."

Having my clothes ripped from my body as we grapple throughout the grocery store…

"I'm stronger than this."

Driving home from brief outings while being assaulted…

"I'm stronger than this."

Sadly, our home was no sanctuary either. And the anxiety I felt transformed into fear. I found myself in a constant state of fear. I feared what Cade would try to do next. I feared for the safety of my wife and our pets. However, despite my staggering angst, I knew that Cade would never hurt his Uncle Brett. Perhaps it was because he knew that there was something special about Uncle Brett. Regardless of the reason, there was always an extraordinary connection between the two of them. My wife and I, on the other hand, were Cade's targets. And there was no telling when he was going to strike next.

Sleep was no longer an option. My adrenaline spiked at the slightest sound. Lying in bed, I gently stroked Julee's head – the spot where her hair was pulled from the roots. My eyes slowly began to close.

"What's that noise?" Prepared to defend myself I jumped to my feet.

"Hey Tramp," I whispered. With his tail wagging, he stood on his hind legs. It's been quite a while since he and Gumbo had gotten any attention. I paused for a moment and cuddled them both on the floor. The remainder of the night was remarkably quiet. Even though I couldn't sleep, I somehow managed to feel rested.

Any amount of rest made going to work the next day a bit easier. The school year had just ended and Julee was taking time off to stay with Cade.

"Call me if you need me," I instructed as I headed out the door.

"I'll be fine," she replied. "I'm just going to get things together for his trip to Camp Sunshine."

A big smile overcame Cade's face as he thought about camp.

Upon my arrival to work I checked in with Julee once more.

"It's a good day," she assured me.

With my best poker face, I walked into the bank. I was able to fool most people with my charming fake smile. Nellie, on the other hand, always knew better. I can't quite explain it. She just knew. Nellie was my guardian angel at work. She had a full head of soft-curled charcoal hair that was roller set at the beauty salon every Thursday afternoon. It was five days since her last set and her perfect ringlets hung in more waves than curls. Her silvery edges danced about her face highlighting her warm brown skin. In addition to working for the bank for over thirty years she was also a pastor of a small church.

"You're looking dapper today Boss!"

"Thanks Nellie. You look nice as well."

"How's my boy?"

"Cade's great."

"Sit down Boss. We're gonna pray on this."

"Everything's fine Nellie," I reiterated.

Doing as her eyes instructed, I sat down and shut up. She extended her hands and we embraced across the desk. The warmth in her touch increased with every spoken word. My eyes remained closed as Nellie continued to pray.

"Thank you Nellie." I looked up towards her and smiled.

"You are very welcome." She replied and continued. "Things are going to be all right. I got a strong feeling about this. Now I ain't saying the devil won't try to distract you. He's sneaky like that. He will try to mock the good that God is doing. Remember everything he does is the opposite of what God does. He will try to take your faith and replace it with fear. He will try to take your peace and replace it with worry. Don't you let him do it. You tell that devil 'Nellie don't play that.' Love you Boss."

"Love you too."

Nellie made life at work a whole lot easier. Later that same day I noticed a missed call from an unknown number and there was a voicemail that was left.

"Hello…I don't know you but your wife asked me to call you. I was driving down the street and she ran up to my car screaming. She said your son was attacking her. She said that she escaped through the bedroom window. She also asked me to get help… I don't know what to do… I guess I will call the police."

The road seemed to stretch longer and longer as I raced home. I pushed my tiny Prius-C to its limits. As fast as I could, I finally made it home. The stranger from my voicemail did as Julee asked and called the police. There were two officers seated at my house when I arrived. Cade and Julee both were unexpectedly calm while speaking with the officers. The men stayed a bit longer and I joined them in the conversation. Before leaving, the officers asked if we planned to press charges. With confusion in our eyes, we glanced towards each other. "No," together we told the officers. Cade is our son and we planned to deal with him even if it killed us.

Things were getting progressively worse and Cade's psychiatrist was no help. I honestly believed that he wanted to help. However, each time I raised concern all he did was change Cade's medication. My gut was telling me that the anti-psychotic drugs were causing Cade's frequent violent attacks. The doctor, on the other hand, believed that because Cade was violent; well, then he needed the medication.

Cade did not attend Camp Sunshine in the summer of 2011. Instead, he was admitted to the adolescent psychiatric unit. We entered through the hospital's emergency room. Cade was out of control. Heartbroken, we watched as the police on duty restrained him. For the safety of the hospital staff, it wasn't long before they sedated him. The weeks he spent in the hospital seemed like an eternity. Visits were tightly supervised as my son was now labeled violent.

It was my first meeting with the hospital's psychiatrist. I informed him of Cade's behavior changes and how I believed that they were related to his anti-psychotic medications. The doctor, of course, did his best to convince me otherwise. He touted his credentials and explained to me that I was merely a parent. Secretly, I wanted to punch him in the mouth. Unfortunately, we already had one violent classification in the family so I just went along. Although I was certain that the medication was the problem, I put my faith in the doctor's hands. I was desperate to get my son back.

The day came for Cade's discharge from the hospital. It was one of the happiest days of my life. It was also one of the scariest. Cade was prescribed a new medication. Despite my concerns, it was still an anti-psychotic drug. I drove home frightened of being attacked while behind the wheel. My fears; however, proved to be unnecessary. Cade did great. We got home and he went straight to his room. Just as he did on any other usual day, he started playing with his toys. Sitting on the couch, I looked over towards Julee. Relieved, we both sighed. The sound of Cade playing was music to our ears.

Abruptly and without warning, the happy sounds were gone.

"I'm the bad guy," Cade groaned in the eeriest of voices.

The next seven days were straight out of a horror movie. Cade's violence was at an all-time high. He broke everything in sight and to make matters worse, he now had insomnia. The violence was 24 hours a day. We slept with the bedroom door locked and a dresser pushed in front of it. I was forced to escort Julee to the bathroom in the middle of the night and to stand guard at the door.

A week later we found ourselves back in the emergency room.

"Get this shit out of his system," I demanded.

The hospital's psychiatrist repeated his stance, "I still don't believe it's the medication. Unfortunately with autism, violence during puberty is a very common occurrence."

Several long term facilities were recommended. The thought of Cade living so far from home was a feeling I will never forget. I informed the hospital staff that I wasn't ready to give up. I also let them know that I wasn't willing to sign a consent form for anymore anti-psychotic drugs. I begged them to try something different. Sitting with the doctor, I promised that if they got the anti-psychotic drugs out of Cade's system they would never see me again. The supervised visits that I had with Cade will remain etched in my mind forever.

Eagerly waiting, I sat at the table. It was a sterile environment surrounded by windows. Staff members stood outside these windows observing the patients' interactions within. Like rodents in a glass tank on a pet store shelf, we knew that we were being watched.

The clock ticked loudly.

My chair gave way as I leaned back to scan the room. The area was reminiscent of a middle school classroom. A series of calendars and maps hung along the one wall that had no windows. There was also a chalk board that was framed upon that same wall. The round tables where visitors sat were industrial in nature and surrounded by yellow and orange plastic chairs.

The clock ticked loudly.

I observed the interactions at the adjacent tables. The other visitors were obviously looking for the same thing as me. They were looking for hope; or at least some remote resemblance of hope.

The clock ticked loudly.

Through the window I saw Cade approach. We sat across from each other and talked about all of his favorite things. It became increasingly harder not to cry. We continued our talk and Cade reached out his hand. For the next several minutes we sat across from each other holding hands. Cade looked me in the eye. And without saying a word he let me know that he was going to be all right. I could feel his sadness and his desire to go home. My worries were suddenly lifted.

The date came for Cade to be discharged from his second hospital stay, but this time it was different. The idea of being attacked while driving didn't even cross my mind. The non-stop violent outbursts stopped when the anti-psychotic drugs stopped. The funny thing is I didn't need a degree to figure that out. I just needed to be a parent. My focus on Cade shifted back to what I believed to be migraines. By tracking his headaches the common triggers were pointing to allergies. Unfortunately, Cade had a different allergy from every season. And although he was no longer violent towards others, he still whacked it to me when his pain got to be unbearable. That part still sucked but I was thankful to be the only person he used as his occasional punching bag.

By observing Cade I began to sense the moments that a headache was approaching. When these subtle clues presented themselves, I gave him an over the counter migraine pill and it actually made a difference. Before long we took a bottle of Excedrine everywhere that we went.

"Cade," I asked. "Where would you like to go for vacation?"

"Disney World and Universal Studios," he shouted in joy. "Go ride *The Mummy*."

So we did, and he's been riding *The Mummy* almost every year since. It's frightening to think about the kids that may be locked up in a facility due to a medication that doesn't agree with them. It's even more frightening to think about these children being forced to take these medications for the rest of their lives.

Chapter 3

Winds of Change

For some reason, I've had a lot of life changing events happen to me in the month of August. It all started August 1996 when I accepted a dreadful job as a department manager for Sears. Since I wasn't an hourly paid employee, I had to work early mornings until late evenings; all for a mediocre salary. My best memory of that job was the time that a gentleman wearing baggy shorts crapped his pants on the escalator. The result was a big mound of shit that reached the second floor. I turned off the escalator and paused for a moment staring at the poop before me. Failing to notice the customer walking up the steps, I stopped him as he approached.

"I apologize for the inconvenience Sir," I informed him. "But I'm going to have to ask that you use the elevator."

"Look, you young punk," he replied. "You should have told me that before I started walking up these damn steps."

Determined to finish his ascent he marched right past me. That final step of his; however, made it all worthwhile.

I hated that crappy job and planned to quit soon after I started. But life had different plans for me. Julee became pregnant and I decided to stay throughout her pregnancy. The following July Cade was born and in August 1997 I started my first job in banking. Seven years later, in August of 2004 I accepted a new job with a competing bank.

However, none of these changes remotely prepared us for what would happen in August of 2005. Strong warnings were issued to residents of the gulf coast region as we braced for Hurricane Katrina.

Don't Squeeze the Spaceman's Taco

August 26, 2005:

"Mr. Kelly," Daniel announced as he skipped down the staircase, "I have to make stinky."

"Dan the man, you know where the stinky room is," I smiled as I watched Daniel make his way to the bathroom.

Daniel was the neighbor's kid. He was happy and hyper. But most importantly, he was Cade's best friend. We became neighbors August 30, 2004. We may have lost our home a year later but in that one year we gained family.

"Mr. Kelly, I ever told you about the time my Katelyn made spaghetti?" Katelyn was Daniel's older sister. Anytime we needed a babysitter Katelyn was always there.

"No Daniel. I don't think that you did."

"This one time my Katelyn was making spaghetti and I was watching Spiderman. Spiderman was fighting the Green Goblin. Did you see that movie? That was a good movie and my Katelyn made spaghetti." Daniel's stories always had the same pattern. There was a beginning, a very long middle and absolutely no ending. Although they never led anywhere, Daniel's stories were definitely entertaining.

"Mr. Kelly," Daniel peeked through the bathroom door. "I'm still making stinky."

That kid always cracked me up. Continuing our conversation, I checked my hurricane supply kit. Certain things were a necessity for life in southern Louisiana. With pen and paper in hand, I checked off my list.

- flash light
- batteries
- pocket knife

- duct tape
- candles / oil lamps
- lighter
- portable radio
- toilet paper
- first aid kit
- insect repellent
- plastic cups caught at a Mardi Gras parade
- snacks
- plastic utensils
- potted meat

And there was one more item that was also needed. Survivors of Hurricane Betsy in 1965 learned that it's a good idea to keep an ax in the attic; just in case the levees fail. With rapidly rising water it may be the only way to escape your home. While making a list of items needed to complete my kit a weather alert flashed upon the TV screen. The National Hurricane Center had just issued an advisory that the storm was predicted to make landfall as a major hurricane.

August 27, 2005:

It was the early morning hours and the New Orleans metro area had just been placed under a hurricane watch. Our hurricane supply kit was fully stocked. A couple hours later my pan was sizzling with left over crawfish from Julee's etouffee. There's nothing like breakfast on the bayou. Cade was eight years old at the time.

"Breakfast is ready," I announced.

With his Ninja Turtle pajamas still twisted from sleeping restlessly, Cade fixed two plates. One for him and one for Manny Bear. Distracting Cade, I stole a few bites of Manny's omelet. The rest of the morning was spent playing with action figures and watching cartoons.

Through the glass of the French doors I glanced out to the back yard. There was a large trampoline that I recently assembled for Cade's birthday. It was just one of the many items we bought hoping that Cade would enjoy. I couldn't get him to play on that damn trampoline for more than thirty seconds. The same was true of his bicycle. Cade made absolutely no attempt to pedal.

"Cade," I asked. "Would you like to go jump on the trampoline with me?"

"No," he answered. "Play toys."

Cade went on playing with his action figures and I finished the rest of the omelet. As I picked up Manny Bear's dirty plate there was a knock on the door.

"Mr. Kelly," Daniel announced as he opened the front door. "Guess what?"

"What?" I questioned.

"I already made stinky this morning and it was green."

"Really?"

"Yeah, and my mom said it was because I ate a green snowball. And then sometime I eat a yellow snowball but it's not yellow. What color stinky do you make?"

"Mostly it's just brown," I replied.

"Just brown?" There was a clear-cut disappointment in Daniel's voice. "You should try making a different color sometime."

"Thank you Daniel. I will keep that in mind."

"Mr. Kelly," again he asked for my attention. "I can run really fast. Remember that time we went running at Chalmette High School?"

"Do you mean yesterday, Daniel?"

"Yeah," he continued with a sense of pride. "And I can run fast. And guess what?"

"What's that Dan the man?"

"And that's not the only time that I ran fast. This one time I ran fast and my friend couldn't catch me. And then we had to go inside because the mosquito truck was coming. The mosquito truck smells yucky. And you know what?"

"What?"

"I can run fast. Hey, can I play on the trampoline with Cade?"

"I don't think Cade wants to play on the trampoline but you can play all you want."

"Hello Cade," Daniel announced as he made his way to the living room. "You want to play on the trampoline?"

Quickly and without hesitation, Cade put down his action figures. The two boys bounced on the trampoline for well over an hour.

"Well look at that," declared Julee. We both watched in awe as they jumped and laughed. It was a warm sunny day in southeast Louisiana. With such beautiful blue skies it was hard to imagine the darkness that was lurking in the gulf.

"Would you boys like a snack?" asked Julee.

"Yeah!" They shouted excitedly.

Cade opted for cookies and Daniel chose his usual favorite – uncooked ramen noodles.

"Mr. Kelly," Daniel questioned. "Did you see how high I jumped?"

"Yeah man. That was fantastic."

"I know," he agreed munching on his crinkly, dry, processed treat. "This one time I was jumping high and my Katelyn was doing her homework. And I was jumping high. You should have seen that. I jumped real high. I think I want to go ride my bike now. You want to watch how fast I can ride my bike?"

"I would love to see that Dan the man." To my surprise Cade pulled out the bike that he never rode and pedaled right beside Daniel. Of course he wasn't as fast as Daniel. But then again, who could possibly be that fast?

Many families in St. Bernard parish were supported by the money they earned from fishing and trawling. Daniel's father was one of the parish's many local fishermen. With the storm approaching it was time to secure his boat. Sadly, play time was coming to an end. Daniel's father walked over and stated that it was time to go.

Squeezing his eyes tightly shut, Daniel assured his father, "I can't hear you and I can't see you either."

Unfortunately, Daniel's father didn't buy into it and the two of them were shortly on their way.

I remember how brightly the stars shone that night. Cade and I lay on the trampoline pointing out various constellations. In the stars Cade could see Spiderman, the Hulk and Captain America. I guess it is a Marvel universe after all. While tucking Cade and Manny Bear into bed a weather update flashed upon the screen. Katrina was now a Category 3 hurricane with maximum sustained winds over 115 mph. The National Hurricane Center has now placed us under a hurricane warning. I did what most residents in the region did that night and slept with one eye open.

August 28, 2005:

It was the wee hours of the morning. Katrina has now strengthened into an extremely powerful and rare Category 5 hurricane. Maximum sustained winds were over 175 mph and the storm was showing no sign of turning away. Local government officials warned of certain death to any resident who failed to evacuate. Our suitcases were filled with a few articles of clothing and the documents that we deemed to be important. As we bid farewell to Daniel and his family, we promised that we'd be back to see each other within a couple days.

Soon after daybreak, we boarded our SUV and thirteen hours later we had only driven ninety miles. Even though all traffic lanes were converted outbound, we were still moving at a snail's pace. The remainder of the day was spent driving along the highways while listening carefully to our radio for critical weather updates. Family and friends followed in cars caravanned behind us.

August 29, 2005:

We finally reached our destination. The approximate 450 mile drive to Hot Springs, AR took us over twenty-three hours. During the grueling drive, there were numerous radio reports of extreme wind, rain and tornadoes ripping right through our neighborhood. Katrina's landfall struck at the heart of St. Bernard Parish. That day we lost more than our home. We lost our entire community.

Sadness overcame me when I realized that we'd be breaking our promise to the neighbors. There was no way that we were going home anytime soon. Praying for the safety and well-being of those that we knew and loved, we anxiously awaited their calls.

Meanwhile, we decided to make the best of our cabin on the lake. Iris' father-in-law Willie and I had a long conversation on a deck overlooking the sparkling clear water. The two of us reminisced about the unique culture of St. Bernard Parish. Giggling and looking mischievous, Cade walked over to join us. Willie spotted a beautiful bird flying by and shared the moment with Cade. To Willie's surprise Cade yelled, "Look out!"

Speaking of himself in the third person, Cade boasted hysterically, "You pushed old man Willie in the water."

A few days later we found ourselves seeking long term refuge. It was over 800 miles to the suburbs of Charlotte, NC. Fortunately, we were no longer in hurricane evacuation traffic. Julee's cousin, Pat and cousin-in-law, Michael were living in the small town of Belmont. After performing his medical residency in Winston Salem, NC, Michael decided to start a family practice in a place that Julee and I referred to as Pleasantville. In Belmont we found peace. The outpouring of love and support was overwhelming. We realized just how fortunate we were as we watched the tragedy unfolding in the Superdome from the comfort of a furnished four bedroom home. The home was offered to us by Pat's friend, Betty.

Betty was a remarkable pioneer spirited woman. A few years earlier, she and her husband Hugh had a log cabin built among fifty secluded wooded acres in nearby Lincolnton. Their former home in Belmont had been listed for sale. So that we'd have a comfortable place to stay, they took their house off the market. Neither of them had ever met us, yet they sacrificed the sale of their home. Numerous times we offered to pay them rent, but they just wouldn't hear of it. As time passed and things began to settle, we realized that we wouldn't be going back to St. Bernard Parish anytime soon. With our credit ravaged from the storm, Betty and her husband, Hugh offered to owner finance the sale of their home to us. Because of their generosity, we were able to get back on our feet in a home where Cade could be as loud as he wanted to be.

It was when we enrolled Cade in a new school that we realized just how easily he dealt with change. We've read countless articles about keeping things routine for children with autism. What good is it to shelter a child from change in an ever changing world? Cade has always been exposed to change. And as a result, he handles it like a champ.

Uncertainty weighed heavily upon us as we dropped Cade off for his first day at his new school. We had no idea if my son would ever see his former classmates from Louisiana again. For a moment, I contemplated shadowing Cade in class for a few days; a sort of *21 Jump Street* style stake out. But I could never pass for a third grader, so we just walked him to the door and said good bye. Upon entering the building, he turned around and waved. "Bye Mom and Dad. Going to school. See you soon."

Shortly after Cade returned to school I returned to work. Being displaced with a banking background, Charlotte was a good place to be. Two things were plentiful in the Queen City -- banks and Bojangles' chicken. Two pieces (spicy) and a biscuit later I started a new job with Bank of America.

It's now eight years later and time to bid my banking job farewell. The hardest part is telling Nellie good bye.

Before leaving I gather my team for a meeting. While everyone is seated I read them one of my mom's poems. Of all her writings this one was the most special to me. Tears flowed as I read the final words on the page. Passing a tissue box, we share one final group hug.

With my desk completely packed, I head for the exit door. "Nellie…" I look her in the eyes.

"Don't you say it Boss," she pauses. "Don't you dare say good bye."

"See you soon."

"That's right Boss. See you soon."

Before driving off, I notice Nellie's head poking out the bank's door.

"One last thing Boss," grinning she continues. "Don't think I ain't mad at you for leaving me here to work with a woman!"

A tremendous sense of freedom takes over me while driving home. Sure, it's worrisome not knowing if I can generate enough money to get by. Nonetheless, I feel remarkably free.

We stand side by side at the kitchen sink that evening, Julee and me. By the time dinner is set, the family is fed and the kitchen is cleaned; it's time to go to bed and do it all over again tomorrow. I wash the dishes and Julee rinses and stacks them on the side to dry. Turning off the water she asks, "So what did they think about your mom's poem?"

"I think they liked it," with a slight chuckle I continue. "They cried like babies."

"What's so funny about them crying?"

Thinking of what Nellie said I smile. "I'll be in the bedroom talking to my mom."

The first thing I notice while walking to the bedroom is Cade's dirty laundry scattered randomly across the hallway floor. It's hard being a neat freak living with Cade and brother-in-law Brett. Neither one has the slightest worry about basic household cleanliness. Sticky handles and dirty knobs are about as predictable as indigestion at a Chinese buffet. Cade is sound asleep so I pick up his dirty clothes and head back towards the laundry room. Making my way down the hallway I hear what sounds like two cats fighting in an alley.

"Brett," I knock on his door. "Would you try not singing so loudly? Cade is sleeping."

"Oh, ok," he replies. "Why? Was I being loud?"

"Just a little." Continuing my way to the laundry room, I close Brett's door. Journey's "Don't Stop Believin'" will never be the same.

The clothes are in the hamper and I walk quietly back to my bedroom. Our walnut floors creak with every step that I make. I stop for a moment to admire Cade's art work. Some of his finest pieces are hung along the walls in our hallway. Periodically we'll change out his collection to make room for his new work. There's one piece, however, that always remains constant. A crayon sketched red house is the first time that Cade called North Carolina home. My fingers tap gently against the rustic wooden frame.

A couple feet away hangs another one of my favorite pieces. It's from one of Cade's back to school classroom assignments. The students were asked to draw pictures of their recent summer vacations. Among the projects submitted were numerous depictions of beaches, carousels and roller coasters. Cade's sketch, on the other hand, was unlike any other. It was a year following Hurricane Katrina and Cade was spending his summer vacation with my sister Iris in Louisiana. Cade's art project showcased my sister's beautiful Colonial style home. His teacher; however, couldn't figure out the large white square on top of two black circles.

"That," I told his teacher, "is the FEMA trailer parked in my sister's front yard."

I go back to my bedroom for my late night chat with Mom. Our bedroom is much like the rest of our house; lost somewhere in the middle of a half-finished renovation. Every time I start a new project, Cade or Brett destroys it. Living with those two has left me with a "why bother" attitude towards home improvement. Our bedroom walls remain bare from where I removed the 1970's patterned wallpaper. I stare for a moment at the one piece of art that we do have on the wall. It's a framed paint-by-numbers version of Thomas Gainsborough's *The Blue Boy*. Julee found this painting a couple months after we arrived in Belmont while shopping at a consignment shop with Betty. As they strolled the endless aisles of antiques, Julee shared the story of a gift that her father once gave to his mother.

Many years ago Julee's father, Brent bought his mother a reproduction of the famous painting. "To Mom. Love Doo," he so lovingly inscribed on the back. Oddly enough I call Cade my "Doo-Doo." Following Julee's father's death, we kept the painting in our attic. It wasn't until we moved to our last home in Louisiana that we actually hung it up. There was a spot in our stairwell that was just perfect for *The Blue Boy*. While gathering our important documents in preparation of our hurricane evacuation, Julee sat in the stairwell facing the painting.

"Please look after our home," she instructed Blue.

In the midst of the storm, the water level rose well into the second floor -- right at Blue's neck to be exact. Blue's eyes remained above the water the entire time. There was a volunteer group from Texas that helped to empty our house following Hurricane Katrina. Stripped down to the bare studs, what made our house a home was now a mountain of debris in the front yard. Everything that we owned was in that pile. Everything except for Blue, that is. For some unknown reason, the group from Texas decided to hang Blue back up in our house. This time he was positioned right at the center of our home, nailed to one of the many exposed studs. Proud of the job that he'd done, I took Blue back to North Carolina with me. Since mold had set into the painting, I had to remove everything that was hanging below the water line. To this day, Blue's head remains prominently displayed framed on a shelf in our living room.

While sharing this story with Betty, the song "My Girl" by The Temptations began airing throughout the store. Brent used to sing this song to Julee whenever she was feeling down. At that moment, Julee looked over towards the speaker and there he was; a crafty do-it-yourself rendition of the same painting. It was like staring at a puppy in a pet store window. Needless to say, Paint-by-Numbers Blue Boy found himself a new home that day.

And tonight I'm sitting right beside Blue as I'm talking to Mom. "I hope that I'm doing the right thing." I continue, "I know that Cade needs me right now." Waiting for her answer, I sigh. "I'm just scared." Bit by bit Mom's words comfort me until eventually I fall asleep. The next morning I wake to her message.

Don't Squeeze the Spaceman's Taco

"Heaven Sent"

His healing grace is all I need
To wash away the pain
A miracle is on the way
He's told me that again
Our mother Dear is watching us
She wants us to be wise
With her there's consolation too
The tears that's in my eyes
I needn't ever be afraid
There's so much to be done
The labor in the vineyards too
The call to everyone
He's there with his rejoicing smile
We come alive each day
The everlasting spring of life
Come see and learn the way

Helen Melerine

Rested from a good night's sleep, I slowly roll over.

"It's 5:00 a.m." Noticing the clock, I ask myself, "Why am I awake?"

The annoying sound of slamming cabinets continues from the kitchen. I peek out the bedroom door and notice Brett walking back to his room. He's wearing his usual nightly attire. His striped tank top is tucked tightly into his smiley face pajama pants. Brett is 6'3" and his pants are pulled so high up to his chest that it has created a very unflattering empire waist / moose knuckle combination. Brett's camelbro's come in many colors. On a tall gentleman, such as my brother-in-law, this undoubtedly also creates a high-water effect. Lucky for me, it better accentuates Brett's striped tube socks and fully laced high top tennis shoes.

Brett has very regimented routines. He wakes up at 5:00 a.m. every morning and makes himself a cup of coffee. Sometime he prepares his coffee at 5:00 a.m. and then goes back to sleep. When Brett doesn't go back to sleep, he gets dressed and heads out on his scooter to the gym. And as far as Brett's concerned, there's no better way to reward yourself for hard work at the gym than by picking up a sausage biscuit, hash browns and large soda. He then takes his food home and changes back into his pajamas. Why? Because according to Brett, "You are supposed to eat breakfast in your pajamas."

In the seventies Brett was diagnosed as emotionally disturbed. However, by today's standards he would be considered to be somewhere along the autism spectrum. Brett is very independent and takes great pride in that. He has never been on government assistance because he chooses to work. Although he is a very dedicated employee, he will never make enough money to fully support himself. Unfortunately, the system chooses to punish people like Brett. We have tried numerous times to get disability benefits for him, but because of his long history of washing dishes he did not qualify. We were told by the Social Security Administration that the only way Brett would qualify would be if something physically happened to his hands that prevented him from washing dishes. Brett works only part time hours and earns minimum wage. However, the job makes him feel good about himself. And that's something that we would never want take away from him anyway. We promised Julee's parents, when they were alive, that we would always look out for Brett.

The sound of running footsteps outside my window lets me know that Brett is on his way to the gym. For some reason, he always runs along the driveway. The time of day or purpose doesn't matter whatsoever. Brett always, and I mean always runs while on the driveway. He keeps his scooter parked in the shed behind our house.

Don't Squeeze the Spaceman's Taco

Brum...brum...brum...

The puny engine whines as Brett zips on by. Unable to fall back asleep, I decide to tend to some much needed yard work. There's a pile of branches that I recently cut down. Those branches, along with other yard waste, need to be hauled away. I start loading my trailer. While carrying the branches past the front corner of the house I notice a familiar sight. One of the landscape lights I recently purchased has been crushed. These lights have been replaced at least three times this summer alone.

For the longest time I was baffled by what kept happening to the lights. And then it hit me. One thing I've learned growing up along the Mississippi River is that it's hard for a large boat to make sudden turns. As Brett runs along the driveway, led by his pudgy belly, he doesn't slow down when reaching the front corner. Therefore, as he steers right to rim the sidewalk he tramples through everything that's within his path. I've been thinking about getting Brett a sign to wear on his rump -- "Wide right turns." Numerous times I've demonstrated slowing down in hopes of saving the lighting and our plants. However, Brett's only response is, "I didn't do it."

Gathering the last of the remaining branches on the ground, I spot Brett returning home from the gym. There's a huge grin stretched all the way across his face.

Driving briskly past me in the yard, Brett shakes his head. "Oooooh!" He exclaims.

From the driveway, I watch Brett park his scooter in the shed behind the house.

"Brett," I ask as he shuts the door behind him, "Would you please help me take these branches to the dump?"

"Oh yeah," he replies. I must admit, Brett is always willing to help whenever asked. "Let me eat my breakfast first."

With a Chick-fil-a bag and extra-large Styrofoam cup in hand, he swiftly runs towards the front of the house. As he turns along what I refer to as Dead Plant's Curve, I could hear him shouting, "I didn't do it!"

I pick up two more landscape lights from the nearby Lowe's that morning. Unlike my usual visits, I'm in and out in no time flat. Home improvement stores can easily get me distracted. Perhaps it's a reminder of the many projects I still have left unfinished.

Returning home I notice Brett through the picture window. That silly grin of his is still plastered across his face. Holding a hot sauce covered biscuit, he gazes out the window. I see him marvel at the birds resting on the playhouse, at the squirrels running across the branches, at the dogs playing in the morning sun. He watches ever so gleefully until he notices me.

"Oooooh!" Shaking his head he continues. "I don't know why you had to come home and ruin my good day."

Brett and I spend much of our time together in fake arguments calling each other made up names. It all started one day when Brett called me a "tote." By the context of the sentence, I knew that a tote was the equivalent of an asshole.

"Shut up you dribble-drot," I announce as I pass him by.

"At least I'm not a jawanna-doob like you."

"What the hell is a jawanna-doob?" I ask.

"Oh...," he pauses for a moment searching the hard drive within his head. "It's a tote."

It's safe to say that the origin of most of Brett's words is derived from the word "tote." He continues his ramblings while he finishes breakfast. Quite naturally, he's redressed in his pajamas of course -- moose knuckle and all.

We take our trip to the dump. By the time we unload the branches and get Brett a caramel Frappuccino, a couple hours have passed. We get home and Cade is now awake. He and Julee are watching Disney's *Aladdin*. Although he has seen the movie many times already, the story continues to intrigue him. There's something magical about a street rat kid becoming a prince and living the life of his dreams. Longing for moments like this, I join the two of them on the couch.

"What would Cade do with three wishes?" I look at him and wonder.

There's a scene in the film where Aladdin and Jasmine share their sentiments of feeling "trapped." I close my eyes and think of what it must be like to be Cade.

"Dad," he asks for my attention. "Who's Aladdin like?"

"I don't know Cade." Opening my eyes, I repeat his question. "Who's Aladdin like?"

"You," he continues speaking of himself in the third person.

"That's right buddy. Aladdin is just like you, Cade."

Chapter 4

Cade-isms

Here's a few facts to consider. According to the Centers for Disease Control and Prevention about 1 in 59 children are identified as having autism spectrum disorder (ASD). With boys the prevalence is four time more common than girls. As of 2005, the average medical cost for children with ASD enrolled in Medicaid was $10,709 per child. Aside from medical costs, treatments such as speech and occupational therapies and other behavioral interventions ranged from $40,000 to $60,000 per year per child. Not to mention the cost of any treatment that the parents may need themselves while dealing with all of this crap. In other words, if you have a child with ASD you will most likely spend your life stressed out and broke.

And that's us in a nutshell, stressed out and broke. In need of alternative ways to earn money, I transfer my retirement funds into a stock trading account. In plain English, I've become a professional gambler. My cell phone remains by my side at all times. Nervously I watch my money go up and down alongside Cade's mood swings.

9:30 a.m. – The opening bell; time to fetch the scraps left by the top one percent of the country. Like a scavenger I search for the slightest bargain.

"Breakfast Dad." Leaning over, Cade taps me on the shoulder.

My stock trading, or as I call it, "online shopping," has to wait. There's a more pressing matter at hand.

"What would you like Buddy?"

"Oatmeal Daddy."

"Oatmeal it is."

Being home with Cade feels remarkably good. With my measuring cup in hand, I'm prepared to make the best bowl of oatmeal ever. A pat of butter, a dash of cinnamon, in goes the dates and slivered almonds.

"Here you go Buddy." I place the bowl in front of him. "Just the way you like it."

"Breakfast tacos Dad."

"Looks like Dad's eating oatmeal," I tell him.

Cade, on the other hand, gets his breakfast tacos. A scoop of salsa, a dollop of sour cream, in goes the cheese and jalapeno peppers.

"Daddy," he asks for my attention. "You don't squeeze the spaceman's taco."

Unexpected laughter sends hot coffee shooting out of my nose. "Why would you squeeze the spaceman's taco?"

"That's not nice," he smiles.

"No," I agree. "That's not nice at all."

"Daddy," again he asks for my attention. "You don't drink the cowboy's orange juice."

The advice that I receive from Cade is priceless. Together, we laugh our way through breakfast. These unique phrases and quotes of his, I refer to as Cade-isms.

"What would you like to do today?" I ask.

"Go to the movies."

Going to the movies is Cade's favorite pastime. We always sit in the first couple of rows near the aisle. There's usually less people there and it makes for an easier exit in the event of a meltdown.

It's a weekday afternoon and there's no need to sit up front. Cade and I are the only ones in the entire theater. Today, we sit wherever we wish. And so we do; the two of us relax a few rows back, right smack in the center. Well, at least Cade relaxes. Me, on the other hand, I'm nervous as heck. Since no one else is in the theater, my phone is resting atop my soda cup. Instead of watching the movie, I'm watching the stock market. My recent stock purchase is sinking and my account balance has dropped five percent since breakfast.

"Oh shit!" I think to myself. "Julee's going to kick my ass."

A few more trades under my belt and I realize that the stock market is a lot like life. Instead of giving up when things turn to shit, you buy in. Stock trading provides me with extra cash as well as daily entertainment. Monday through Friday, my life is a combination of fatherhood, stock trading, cooking, cleaning and listening to Brett's God awful karaoke.

My first month home, I scrub the entire house from floor to ceiling. We have two dogs; a Schnorkie (Schnauzer / Yorkie mix) named Tramp and a Golden Retriever named Gumbo. Tramp doesn't make much mess other than emptying the waste baskets every time we leave the house. Apparently, he gets pissed off when he's left behind. Gumbo, on the other hand, sheds so much that he leaves what looks like tumbleweeds rolling down the hallway. I sweep and vacuum, but the next day they roll back in. By the end of the month Gumbo gets his first crew cut.

My second month home, I organize my chores so they're not overwhelming. I learn to tackle the house one day at a time and one room at a time. My most dreaded day of the week becomes bathroom day -- the day where I repeatedly ask myself, "How the hell did Brett get shit way over there?"

With our new budget constraints, eating out becomes limited. It's time for me to learn how to cook. I grab one of Julee's cookbooks as tears run slowly down my cheeks. My eyes close and the salty taste edges the corner of my mouth. Although I hate performing the task at hand, I know that it must be done. With my head turned slightly sideways, I continue until the onion is finely chopped. Meals that I cook come from easy to follow recipes. I'll be the first to admit that I'm a terrible chef. However, I can at least follow instructions. Being married twenty-three years has taught me how to do that quite well. The thing that I've learned about cooking is that once the chopping and dicing is done, the rest is fairly simple. Prep work is the key to a successful meal.

The oven is set to 425 degrees and in goes my casserole dish. Watching shows on the Food Network I've often wondered, "Who cleans up all the mess?" Emeril just cuts it up, throws it in a pan and "Bam!" it's done. The kitchen is left spotless. I don't know what I'm doing wrong because, "Damn!" The clean-up is a nightmare. According to the recipe the dish should be ready in about an hour. Prepared to take on the wreckage, I grab my apron from the hook in the laundry room. The apron was a gift from my dear cousin Pat. Pat gave me this apron as a source of inspiration after quitting my job. It's made of stain resistant fibers and dark blue in color. The apron has a very nice fit to it and it's inscribed with a personal message – "Kitchen Bitch." I turn on some tunes, grab a scrubbing pad and start cleaning.

A voice shrieks from the living room. Removing my headphones, I listen to what's taking place.

"Shut up you son of a bitch!" Cade shouts. "I'm trying to save the world."

Laughing quietly so not to be heard, I tiptoe across the room to get a better look. Cade's playing with his new superhero action figures.

"Lay down and die you piece of shit." His playtime continues. There's no doubt he's enjoying his new toys. Cade has hundreds of action figures and I often question buying new ones. After watching him play today, I will buy him hundreds more. My buddy is very fond of superheroes and through fantasies he can do anything. Although Cade may never save the world, I do believe that he can change it. With Cade as the hero and me as his sidekick, that is our mission.

Granted, Cade was never bitten by a radioactive spider. And when exposed to gamma rays we've always worn protective gear. He's more like one of the X-Men. For those unfamiliar with the X-Men, they're a team of mutants. Mutants are born with superhuman powers because of a gene mutation. Due to fear and prejudice from the so-called "normal" humans, mutants face a constant struggle for peace and acceptance.

We've always been believers of inclusion with Cade. There's so much to experience in this world. It would be foolish to let one, two, three, four or five bad experiences keep us from enjoying life. Despite the fact that Cade carries action figures with him or an occasional plush toy, he's still a teenage boy. Therefore, he enjoys many of the same things as other teenage boys. I feel that it's important for Cade to interact with typical teenagers. And I also feel that it's equally important for them to interact with him. It's the only way to better understand and appreciate each other. I know many parents of children with disabilities that avoid social outings over fear of possible meltdowns. We have left many public places with my shirt ripped off, my pants in shreds and one shoe missing. But we've also left these same places with genuine smiles on our faces and wonderful memories in our hearts.

When venturing out, we always take other people's enjoyment into consideration. For instance, Cade loves restaurants. While dining out, we sit in the least crowded area. If seated at a booth or table we place Cade in the spot furthest from the next guest. He's usually good but he may start stimming and making noise. In that event we're brief and take our orders to go. Hopefully, the other guests stick around long enough for dessert. I hear the tiramisu is off the chain.

It's not unusual for us to receive stares when Cade's behaving "oddly." I understand the curiosity. And while many people are empathetic, some are just plain cruel. It all comes down to getting to know each other before casting judgement. A trip that Cade and I made to Carowinds was a big reminder of this.

It was a breezy summer day at the local amusement park, but nonetheless it was hot. Water sprayed gently across our faces while oscillating fans blew mist into the crowd. The $6.00 sodas were refreshing as we slowly cooled in line. Cade loves roller coasters and this was one of the best in the park. He was fourteen years old, carrying a Cabbage Patch Kid and having the time of his life. We waited behind a group of teens wearing matching t-shirts. It wasn't long before one of the teens spotted Cade's doll. Soon they were pointing, laughing and making ugly faces. Looking towards them, I read their shirts.

"I don't know what they're teaching you at the Joyful Christian Summer Camp but I sure hope this isn't it." Driving my point, I asked, "What would Jesus do?"

A few minutes later we reached the boarding gate and Cade, his Cabbage Patch Kid, the Joyful Christian Summer

Campers and I boarded the train. We laughed. We screamed. We realized that we're not so different after all.

It's time for us mutants to come out of hiding. Cade doesn't have adamantium metal claws. Nor does he have laser beam eyes. His special power is the ability to light up a room through a belly rolling laugh. Additionally, his photographic memory is absolutely mind blowing. Armed with personality, we're set out to prove ourselves to the human world.

    To better fit in with the "normal" humans we've had to improve Cade's communication skills. This we did; however, in a rather unconventional manner. It all started with Cade's first session of speech therapy when he was just four years old.

"Cade," queried his therapist, "can you show me which one is the goat?"

    Overlooking the plastic animals displayed before him, Cade scanned the office. His eyes shifted about the many objects within the room. He had no interest in this so-called goat. A familiar rustling sound brought his attention back to the table. Lying near the herd of collectible wildlife was an opened bag of Cheetos. Tempted by the cheesy morsels Cade reached towards the bag.

    "No Cade." Pulling back the snack sized pouch, his therapist continued. "You must first show me which one is the goat."

    Knowing what was at stake, Cade immediately picked the bearded member of the Bovidae family – the goat.

"Very good Cade. You earned a Cheeto." Cade finished his treat and was ready for more. With the bag of crunchy goodies held high, his therapist presented a new question. "Where is the giraffe?"

Without hesitation Cade grabbed the animal to the far left.

"No Cade. That is a horse." Again his therapist asked, "Where is the giraffe?"

Moving quickly, he made another selection.

"No Cade. That is a camel." This time she did the unthinkable. Removing a bite-sized puff, she ate the Cheeto herself. Licking the powdered cheese from her fingertips, she asked him once more, "Where is the giraffe?"

Appalled by what just happened, Cade gave some thought to his next selection. Carefully he browsed the assortment of plastic animals. "Giraffe!" He shouted as he proudly displayed the long-necked terrestrial creature. Cade and his therapist continued and within no time the bag of Cheetos was emptied.

In addition to "Cheetos" therapy, I started narrating my every move.

"I am holding my toothbrush…"

"I am squeezing the toothpaste…"

"I am brushing my teeth."

This narrative speech became a way of whistling while I worked. Day after day our house was filled with relentless chatter -- sort of like the lyrics to an R. Kelly song. Little by little; however, Cade began to understand when to use certain words.

"I am placing the omelet on the plate…"

"I am carrying the plate…"

"I am walking to the table…"

"Here's your breakfast buddy." Handing him a utensil I continued, "And here is a fork."

Looking up Cade gave me a heartfelt, "Hakuna matata."

"Wow Cade! Hakuna matata. That means 'no worries'."

"For the rest of your days," he excitedly finished the next line.

And for the rest of the morning we hung out at the breakfast table quoting *The Lion King*. Cade has always had a fondness for Disney movies. Watching movies was also a way to increase his vocabulary. Granted, there may not always be an opportunity to discuss regaining control of the Pride Lands from your sinister uncle, but there is always an opportunity to connect.

Deep down we all have a desire to connect. At times, I wish that I was more into sports. I see the passion when fans converse. Truth being, I'm just not that into it. With that being said, I still use whatever knowledge I have of the game just to take part in the discussion.

Good or bad, words are wondrous. They have the power to guide, calm, hurt, astound, humble and bewilder. If Cade was able to add to his arsenal of words by watching movies, why not expand his movie selection? Streaming services offered a boundless library of films. The only thing missing was the popcorn. With our snack bowls filled we embarked on a movie watching marathon.

Lucky for me, Cade was into more than just kids' films. We both enjoyed a good spy movie. Aside from Austin Powers, James Bond was his favorite secret agent. Hence, 007 has taught Cade a number of debonair lines. Not only will this help him when conversing with the ladies, but also when ordering a martini. I don't recall how many times Cade and I watched the *X-*

Men movies together. But I do recall his many inappropriate uses of, "I'm the Juggernaut, bitch!" Be that as it may, the Juggernaut had nothing on Samuel L. Jackson. And before long Cade was randomly shouting, "I have had it with these mother fuckin' snakes on this mother fuckin' plane!"

When Cade was younger he used to simply repeat the last word that we said. His therapist referred to this as echolalia. For instance:

Q. "Cade, would you like a cheeseburger or chicken nuggets?"
A. "Chicken nuggets."

If we changed the question to:

Q. "Cade, would you like chicken nuggets or a cheeseburger?"
A. "Cheeseburger."

By repeating the last option, Cade truly had no choice. And going through life without the ability to choose would just plain suck. Therefore, we began using open ended questions instead. For example:

Q. "Cade, what would you like for dinner?"
A. "Food."
Q. "What kind of food?"
A. "Let's see, um…pizza."

Open ended questions weren't just limited to junk food.

Q. "What do you want to do today?" I waited for his reply.
A. "Watch a movie."

Cade flipped through his DVD collection. It was a midweek afternoon and we would be watching *Shrek* for the tenth or eleventh time. In many ways Cade and I were a lot like the duo from the film. He was the big, misunderstood green guy and I was his loyal companion. Cade inserted the disc and anxiously stood beside the TV. His hand was raised just slightly above the screen.

"What are you doing?" Playfully I asked.

There was a bit of mischief in Cade's eyes; sort of like the time when he pushed old man Willie into the water.

"What are you doing?" Again I asked.

Just then, the DreamWorks logo appeared on the screen. It's an image of a boy sitting on a crescent moon while holding a fishing pole in his hands. Swiftly, Cade drew his hand back and smacked the TV screen.

"Daddy, the DreamWorks fisher boy…" Bursting with laughter, he continued. "Slap that bitch off the moon!"

Not knowing how to respond, I buried my head into the sofa cushion. I too began cracking up. That's when Cade came over and sat next to me on the couch. There was a stain on his new Wolverine t-shirt.

"What's that?" I pointed to the stain.

'Ooh…" Speaking of himself in the third person Cade confessed, "You ate Uncle Brett's candy."

Brett always kept treats hidden within his room. From Pop Tarts to cookies to Peeps bought at an after Easter sale; Cade knew that rummaging through Brett's room was like a trip to Willy Wonka's factory.

"Why did you eat Uncle Brett's candy?" I asked.

"Ooh…that's not nice." He replied.

"No," I tell him. "That's not nice at all. And why did you hit the DreamWorks fisher boy?"

Attempting to hold a straight face, I looked towards him. Rather than answer my question, he laughed. An uproaring, magical laugh that resonated from his core. It was the most enchanting thing that I had ever heard. From his belly, the hysteria continued.

"Daddy," he caught his breath. "Slap that bitch off the moon!"

We both continued laughing long after his bitch slapping stopped.

"Cade," I gave him a fist bump. "You're my best buddy."

When I was Cade's age I had friends that came over nearly every day. The last time Cade had a friend visit was over eight years ago in Louisiana – the day that Daniel marveled over making a green stinky. Our home in North Carolina isn't in a usual neighborhood setting. We live along a busy street on an acre lot in an area of town that has no sidewalks.

I remember the things that I did in my old neighborhood as a teenager. Sneaking out of the house while my parents were sleeping was always an adventure.

"Hey Chucky." I'd knock on the neighbor's window.

Pulling back the sword-like leaves of the Yucca plants along his sill, Chucky would make his escape. Together we'd walk to the nearby convenience store. We knew that if the right clerk was working, we'd be going home with a bottle of Boone's Farm Strawberry Hill or Mad Dog 20/20.

It was a low income neighborhood. Although we were poor, I never really knew it. Or maybe I just blocked it out. While I knew that we couldn't afford the things that my friends' families had, I never considered us to be poor. After all; we lived in a brick house, my father drove a fairly reliable car and we always had a freezer full of shrimp.

The subdivision was filled with families just like mine. It was mostly hard working people with big hearts and little wallets. At least those were the ones that I cared to know. The rest of the neighborhood was comprised of poor white trash that snickered every time Pookie came to visit.

"Look who's coming to play with the white kids," they'd sneer.

Pookie was my best friend. The two of us met in math class. I excelled in algebra and let's just say that Pookie didn't. I remember the day that we met like it was yesterday.

"Hey…" I felt a gentle tap upon my back. "What's the answer to number 3?"

Aside from his dripping Jheri curl, the most noticeable thing about Pookie was his smile. He had a smile that started and ended in dimples the size of New Orleans Garden District potholes. Pookie was several inches taller than me and claimed to be from the hood. However, there was nothing hood-like about this guy. His style was a post-Thriller era Michael Jackson. To keep his skin from getting too ashy, he kept a bottle of lotion in his back pack at all times.

Without saying a word, I slid my paper into view. From the sound of his grinding eraser, Pookie needed help with more than just number 3.

"Thanks for helping me out," leaving the classroom he introduced himself. "I'm Marcel. People call me Dwayne, but my friends call me Pookie."

"Nice to meet you, Pookie. I'm Kelly. Some people call me Jude. But mostly people just call me Kelly."

"How do you get Jude from Kelly?"

"Jude is my middle name, as in St. Jude. We're Catholic and my mom just has a thing for St. Jude I guess. How do you get Pookie from Marcel or Dwayne?"

"You see," he continued. "My mom used to call me Pookie Bear. One day my friends heard her and I've been Pookie ever since."

The following weekend Pookie came over for his first algebra lesson.

"Wow," he exclaimed. "It's doesn't smell like a white person's house in here."

"Thank you?" I questionably replied.

"I mean it smells good. Most white people's houses just smell like Pine Sol."

"Well my mom fried chicken." To avoid sounding as if I were stereotyping, I continued. "It's not because I had a black friend coming over. It's just because she fried some chicken."

It was a crisp autumn Sunday afternoon and that meant only one thing at my house -- football. My dad usually had more than one game going at a time. I think he may have helped pioneer technological advances in television.

Take remote control, for instance: "Kelly, come change the channel."

Then there was his breakthrough with picture in picture: Dad stacked our small portable black and white TV on top of our large wood-grain Zenith console television. There was a different game playing on each device.

The New Orleans Saints game that was taking place in the Superdome that day wasn't being televised. Therefore, Dad had the Saints game resonating from the portable AM radio that was sitting on top of his lap.

Loaded up on football and fried chicken, it was time to study. Pookie still wasn't ready to accept algebra and didn't believe me when I informed him that I used it every day.

"Why the hell would anybody add letters?" he questioned. "It just doesn't make sense."

"If it was just about adding letters then it wouldn't make sense," I agreed. "But check out the first problem on the page: $3x+2=20$. You said your cousin Rodney likes to smoke weed. Right?"

"Yeah. He's a pot head and I know damn well he ain't adding no letters."

"No. But what if you let Rodney borrow $20 and he bought enough weed to roll 3 joints and has $2 left over?"

"I know better than to lend Rodney money."

"Let's just say you did."

"But I didn't."

"OK. Let's just say I loaned Rodney the money." I tried changing the scenario.

"You ain't never seeing that money again."

"I know. I learned my lesson and I will never do it again." I go on to explain. "But, I did it this one time and Rodney bought enough weed to roll 3 joints and he still has $2 left over. You see, 3x+2=20. Using algebra I would subtract 2 from both sides. This leaves me with 3x=18. If I now divide both sides by 3, I get x=6. Therefore, I just used algebra to discover that Rodney paid $6 for each joint that he rolled."

At that moment, a light bulb flashed inside Pookie's head. "Now why didn't Mr. Stutts ever explain it like this in class?"

It's sad to think that Cade may never have a Pookie in his life. However, he's got me and I will be his best friend until the end. With a bucket of crayons, we go on to sketch portraits of each other.

"Wow Cade!" I exclaim. "That's a great drawing of Daddy. But why is my head so square? I look like Frankenstein."

"Daddy," he continues. "You can't go in the sewer because you might get poo in your mustache."

"I'll remember that," I tell him. "And I will try to stay out of the sewer."

Cade finishes his masterpiece by writing the word "Daddy" below the picture. Cade's handwriting is large and barely legible. Letters overlap and some are written backwards.

Cade loves drawing pictures at the beginning of every month. The pictures that he draws are things that he associates with the corresponding month. Not for the month that we're in, mind you, but for the month ahead. Calendars in our home are always set one month into the future. That's the way that Cade likes it. In June, for instance, Cade draws pictures of things associated with July. All the calendars in the house are then switched to July.

His artwork is abstract to say the least. However, with a little imagination, the pictures come to life. July's artwork usually consists of things such as fireworks, birthday cakes and water slides.

"Cade." Holding a handful of smashed crayons I ask, "Would you like to go buy some new crayons?"

"Yes," he replies. "Come on Tony," he beckons to his cousin. "Let's go to Walmart."

We have two nephews; Darrin and Tony, both in their twenties spending some time with us. They are Cade and Brett's closest friends and for that I love them even more.

Walking through the parking lot we notice a disturbance near the store's entrance. There's a gentleman pinned against a police vehicle with several officers surrounding him.

"Ooh!" Cade shouts. "You see that man by the police car? He's going to jail."

"Shhh…" I do my best to keep Cade quiet.

With his face pressed against the hood of the vehicle, the suspect looks over.

"Ooh!" Again Cade shouts. "That man is going to jail. He got bit by a raccoon."

In unison, the officers glance towards us as well.

Loudly Cade continues rambling. "The police are going to take that man to jail. They're going to lock him up in a cage and HE'S GOING TO DROP THE SOAP!"

Chapter 5

Cover up your Hoo-Ha

"Nice pubes!" Tony jokingly exclaims as Cade walks naked through the hallway. Cade's feeling fresh and clean strutting carefree with his towel in his hand.

"Cover up your hoo-ha," Cade tells himself. "Nobody wants to see your privates. That's weird."

Teaching a child with autism about sexuality can be quite challenging. Sex is a very delicate subject that evokes a whole slew of emotions. I recall my younger self sitting through sex education class in high school giggling every time the words penis and vagina were used. Who am I kidding? I still giggle. There are countless aspects of sex that I need to address with Cade. However, the two most concerning matters are safety and social appropriateness. Don't get me wrong. I truly believe that he needs to learn about manscaping. I hate that he has to search for a needle in a hay stack every time that he goes to the bathroom. However, I'm glad that he knows to lock the stall in a public restroom. He hasn't quite grasped the idea of locking the main door when using a single restroom. I'm still working on that. I'm also working on him not dropping his pants to his knees while using a public urinal. "Just the front Cade. Just the front," I explain as I lift his pants to cover his rump.

Cade attends a school for children with developmental disabilities. There are very limited programs in his school to teach him about sex and sexuality. Unfortunately, sex education is a missing component in much of the special education network. Cade takes everything literal so "spanking the monkey" means just that. And teaching him about "the birds and the bees" means tutoring him on flying creatures. I have to be very concise and use words such as penis, vagina and hoo-ha. It's easy to assume that he will be innocent forever. But that type of thinking can lead to great risks.

Our first lesson on appropriateness with Cade was "No Naked Time in Public." At one point Cade's streaking was spreading faster than the herpes epidemic of the late 1980's. Here's what the streaking phase looked like.

It was a hot Monday afternoon. We were traveling west along Interstate 10 following an extended weekend trip to the Florida Gulf Coast. Cade was just a toddler at the time and still wearing diapers.

"We should stop for something to eat." Julee suggested. "It's almost noon and Cade is probably getting hungry."

"OK," I replied. "There's a McDonalds at the next exit. Cade can run through the play area and get the wiggles out of his system."

A bit tired from our days on the beach, we ordered our food and sat in the enclosed playground. Cade, on the other hand was fascinated by the vibrant colors and assorted textures. I removed his shoes and he began exploring.

"Oooh!" he exclaimed as he entered the bright red tube.

Sounds of wonderment echoed as he crawled his way through the plastic maze. Before long a young girl joined in on the fun.

"I'm a princess," she proclaimed as she kicked off her Little Mermaid sneakers.

Her feet drug along the ground causing her hair to rise with static.

"Look at my hair mom," she shouted.

Bouncing and giggling she made her way to the tube entrance. Her Ariel impersonation was spot on. She began singing "Part of Your World" as she flapped her fins through the tunnel.

"Hey," the singing paused. "Somebody's socks."

A bit taken aback, she resumed her singing as the journey continued.

"Mom! Somebody left their pants in here."

There was no telling what treasures awaited the young princess.

"And a shirt too!"

From the bottom I heard Cade's voice as he prepared for his exit down the slide. The singing mermaid wasn't far behind.

"Ewww!" She yelled out in disbelief. "Somebody's diaper!"

Inch by inch Cade's tush scooted down the slide. The fairy tale was over. The mermaid princess transformed into a sea witch and she back tracked her way out of the maze.

"I will not go down a butt slide!"

I am pleased to say that the public streaking stopped years before Cade developed a hairy hoo-ha. His streaking is now limited to the interior of our home. But; as most parents know, when one phase ends another one begins. It's like that spinning carnival ride that makes you dizzy and a bit nauseous. You're glad when it's finally over. Then, as you're breathing a sigh of relief, the attendant announces that there's no one else in line and gives you another run.

An "eclipse" – that's what we call the moment when a new phase overlaps an old one? During one of Cade's many eclipses, the naked phase was crossing over the chocolate phase. During the chocolate phase, Cade used the word "chocolate" to express excitement. If I threw him a ball, for instance, he would shout, "Get the chocolate ball!" There was nothing chocolate about the ball, mind you. Not the color nor even the taste. Here's what that eclipse looked like.

It was a usual summer day in New Orleans. In other words it was hot and muggy. I watched the hanging moss shifting in the wind as I pondered what to do.

"How about the wave pool?" I thought to myself.

Although I have never visited, the wave pool was near the office where I worked. Soon we were on our way. Perspiration drenched our clothing as we entered through the gate. Of the many guests in attendance, we were the only Caucasians. Slathered in sunblock, we were ready to jump in and cool off. Ridding himself of his clothing, Cade immediately streaked across the deck.

"Go in the chocolate pool!" He shouted repeatedly. "Go in the chocolate pool!"

Although awkward at first, we were soon splashing and laughing with everyone else.

I am thankful that the chocolate phase has come and gone. However, guests at our house may still spot the bushy eagle's nest drifting amid the hallways. Be that as it may, I am confident that the majestic bird will one day be confined within the walls surrounding our bathroom. I have managed for him to limit other activities to the bathroom. So I know that I can manage this as well.

It's a peaceful Saturday afternoon. Cade is in the bathroom and I step outside onto the back porch. My eyes close as I inhale the cool autumn air. The vibrant fall colors have mesmerized me ever since moving to the Carolinas. Down on the bayou, there were only two seasons; summer and not summer. During the not summer months the weather changed from hot to cold and back again in an instant. It was the time of the year that Mother Nature shared her hot flashes with the Crescent City region.

Before long Cade joins me outside. Together, we sit down on the cooled red brick steps. With half a piece of baklava in his hand, Cade takes a bite.

"Daddy," he queries. "Who eats baklava?"

"I think you do, buddy."

"Daddy," again he queries. "Who eats baklava?"

"Who buddy?"

"Aladdin."

Cade has always associated food items with various characters. Doing so, he compares himself with those characters.

Pointing to the squirrel climbing down the playhouse he asks, "Daddy, what do squirrels eat?"

"Acorns," I reply as we watch the furry little creature.

Confused, Cade drops his treat. I lean over to reach for an acorn and Tramp races by to finish Cade's crumbs. You can't blame the dog. After all, Aunt Delores makes the best baklava.

Delores is Julee's great aunt. She's a feisty Lebanese woman that says whatever pops into her mind. With her pin curled silver hair, she looks the same as she did the day that I met her over twenty-five years ago. I've always enjoyed my conversations with Aunt Delores. I especially enjoy our conversations during the Easter holiday. This is the time of year that we talk about "cock."

Aunt Delores loves to eat "cock" and quite frankly, she doesn't care who knows about it. In all fairness, "cock" is a Lebanese date cake. The correct spelling is kaak. However, Delores grew up in the south so kaak was pronounced "cock." And Aunt Delores isn't the only "cock" eater in the family. I remember the first time I met Julee's grandmother.

"Johnny gave me some good cock last night." I overheard my future grandmother-in-law raving to Julee's mom.

"Wow," I expressed to Julee. "Your grandmother is really cool."

"I just love Johnny's cock," Maw-Maw Anna continued. "It's not too sweet. It's always just right."

Soon after, Maw-Maw Anna offered to share Johnny's cock with me. Still a bit concerned, I declined her offer. After all, I didn't know Johnny that well yet.

Before long; however, curiosity got the best of me. And when no one else was looking, I nibbled at Johnny's cock. Maw-Maw Anna was right. Johnny's cock was out of sight.

Fortunately for me, kaak is a family tradition. Every year on Good Friday, the ladies on Julee's side of the family get together and roll the "cock." Perhaps it's the kid in me that giggled during sex education class, but I still enjoy a good "cock" story.

Smiling from memories of last Easter, I look down towards Cade. His wrinkled forehead tells me that he's still a touch confused. I explain the reason that squirrels eat acorns and then Cade just starts laughing. That's when I notice Tramp humping Cade's leg.

"What's Tramp doing?" Cade laughs.

Apparently baklava gets Tramp in the mood.

"Stop that," I shout. "You dirty dog."

"Daddy," again Cade asks as I pull the dog away. "What's Tramp doing?"

Suddenly, I have some questions of my own.

- "How do I explain humping?"
- "Does it always make one a dirty dog?"
- "If not, when is it OK to hump?"

Explaining such things to a typical child is challenging enough.

- "How can I explain these things to Cade?"

"Tramp is rubbing his hoo-ha," I explain. "And that's ok. However, you should never rub your hoo-ha on someone else's leg."

Unless, of course, it's two adults and the other person says it's all right to rub your hoo-ha on their leg. But that's another topic that I'm not prepared to discuss.

"Can you play with your hoo-ha outside?" I ask.

"No," he replies. "That's privates."

Cade gets "private" and "privates" mixed up, but either way makes sense. The point is that I want him to know that playing with his privates is something that must be done in private. Humping is a form of masturbation and I want Cade to know that masturbation is a normal and natural thing. However, I do also want him to know that masturbation in public is something that is reserved for a select few freaks in society. I certainly don't want to give Cade the same lecture that my grandmother gave to me.

I was fifteen years old at the time. Lying in bed, I was thinking about a movie that I watched on Cinemax the night before. The channel was scrambled, so I had no idea what the film was about. All I remembered was *squiggly line, squiggly line, boob...squiggly line, squiggly line, boob*. A shake at the door knob quickly interrupted my train of thought.

"Mémère Mary?" I quickly turned and faced the wall.

"Boy what are you doing with that devil in your hand?" She asked in a demanding tone.

Mémère Mary was my grandmother on my mom's side of the family – the Cajun side. I really didn't know how to answer her question. Shamefully, I just stared at the wall as she continued to preach.

"Don't you know that's the devil making you do those things?"

My grandmother's sermon continued for a good ten minutes before her fuzzy slippers went clopping off into the distance.

"Helen," I heard her call out to my mother. "Don't you know I caught that boy with the devil in his hands?"

Embarrassed by the whole ordeal, I remained silent around my mom and grandmother for the next several weeks. My grandmother had the most beautiful crystal blue eyes. It was quite a while before I could look her in those eyes once more.

A couple days later Pookie came over. No Algebra lesson this time. He just came to hang out. It was early in the morning and Mémère Mary was still asleep. She was staying with us until she saved enough money to fix her septic tank at home.

Pookie and I were taking turns playing *Simon*. Although it was Pookie's turn, I watched and listened as the lights changed colors. As the game progressed, the lights changed faster. With each flashing light, the beeping noise intensified. However, lurking between those rapid beeps was a sound that I was dreading -- Mémère Mary's fuzzy slippers were getting closer and they were now in the next room.

"You know," I signaled to Pookie. "We should go hang outside for a while."

"No," he insisted. "I'm getting good at this."

Suddenly, my grandmother's slipper clopping was accompanied by her signature passing of gas. Knocking the game out of Pookie's hands, I reached for the door.

"Where you going boy?" She asked.

It was too late. My grandmother had made her grand entrance.

"I thought I heard someone knocking." I told her.

"I didn't hear anything," Pookie asserted.

"I didn't hear anything either," agreed Mémère Mary. "What's your name baby?"

"My name is Marcel. People call me Dwayne. But my friends call me Pookie."

"Wait a minute," my grandmother continued. "Don't you stay behind Our Lady of Lourdes church in Violet?"

Before long, the two of them were engaged in an hour long conversation. Smiles beamed from their faces as they talked about the people that they both knew. My grandmother rarely left the house yet she knew half the residents of St. Bernard Parish. Once I discovered that the girl I was dating was my cousin after introducing her to my grandmother. I guess that was a good intervention.

"It was so nice meeting you Pookie," she gave him a kiss on his cheek.

Walking away, Mémère Mary reached into the bosom of the pastel colored house dress that she had been wearing for the past three days. It was a loose fitting frock with varying shades of pink, blue and yellow in a crossing vertical and horizontal pattern. There were two front pockets made of the same material but positioned in diagonal patterns. Delighted, she pulled her pack of Bugler roll-your-own tobacco from the left cup of her brassiere. Lightly, she patted both of her breasts. From her right cup, she removed the accommodating rolling papers. My grandmother started smoking when she was just fourteen years old. I haven't seen rolling skills like hers outside of a Cheech & Chong movie. As her slippers clopped towards the back door, one last granny fart was set adrift.

"Yuck!" I held my nose in disbelief.

"Look boy…" She sparked the flint wheel of her slim model Zippo lighter. "Them farts don't pay no rent…" Pausing, she took her lightup drag. "So they got to get out."

"Sorry Pookie." I apologized for my grandmother's flatulence.

"Man your grandmother is great."

"Yeah, but the farting is a little embarrassing. One time she farted while singing 'Happy Birthday' to me. She called it my '21 gun salute.'"

Pookie and I spent the remainder of the morning sharing our embarrassing grandmother stories.

"Just the other day…" Pausing to catch my breath from laughing, I continued. "My grandma caught me choking the chicken in my bedroom."

Pookie's Jheri curl bounced as he whipped his head in complete shock. "That couldn't have been as bad as the time you had the tic on your penis."

"Wait!" I asked with caution. "How did you know about that?'

"Everybody knows about the boy with the tic on his dick." Just when I thought it couldn't get any worse, Pookie added, "My aunt that works in the school cafeteria told me about that a long time ago. Yesterday, when I told her I was coming over she said, 'I know him. That's that little white boy I told you about with the tic on his ding-ding.'" And when I thought it couldn't get any worse than that, he continued. "Now, didn't your sister pull it off with some tweezers?"

Suddenly, Mémère Mary's gas was no longer an embarrassment.

I miss my grandmother and think of her often. Some days I swear that I can smell her. It's funny the way memories trigger our senses. Simple things still remind me of her. Carrying an old metal rake from the shed, I reflect upon late summers with Mémère Mary. Slowly, I comb the back yard. The rake's rusted tips drag along the ground. With continued strokes the leaves pile higher. The large oaks provide a shady space where Tramp and Gumbo love to lie.

Drifting back to my childhood, I'm cooled by the shade of Mémère Mary's mulberry tree.

"Pick the dark purple ones," she would instruct. "The good ones have red specks on them. Those are the sweet ones."

Carefully I'd search. Mémère Mary was making a cobbler and picking the right berries was an important part of the process. I continued until half my Schwegmann's Grocery Store bag was filled.

My precise berry picking was worth all of the painstaking effort. Mémère Mary may have been a lousy cook. But, man she made a mean cobbler.

Scooping the last bit of leaves in my yard, I lick my lips. I can still taste the sweetness of those red-speckled mulberries. Swirling my rake the same way I swirled my spoon, I envision the wine colored juices weaving throughout the sweetened condensed milk.

"Cade," I call out closing the back door behind me. "Let's go to the store. I feel like eating cobbler."

"Daddy," Cade inquires. "Who eats cobbler?"

There was something different that I noticed as Cade exited naked from the bathroom. And that's when it hit me.

"It looks like the jungle brush has been bulldozed." Proudly I ask. "Cade, did you shave your junk?"

"Yes!"

"Well, what did you use?" I ask.

"A hoo-ha razor."

In tears of laughter, I reach for my wallet. It's an old beat up bi-fold. The leather is worn and there are threads hanging at the corners. That's one of the ways that men are different than women. While Julee has over a dozen purses to choose from, one wallet works best for me. The light colored leather is stained from my indigo jeans. It's flattened in the middle and molded to the shape of my butt. I make a list and we head out to find the ingredients for Mémère Mary's cobbler recipe.

"Degree deodorant!" Cade shouts holding up the plastic tube at Target.

"Yes Cade," I acknowledge. "That's Degree deodorant."

"Daddy," he continues. "What kind of deodorant does Superman use?"

"Degree?" I answer with a question.

"Yeah," he confirms. "Degree deodorant... Daddy, what kind of deodorant does Batman use?"

"Degree?" Again I answer in uncertainty.

"Daddy," Cade repeats his question. "What kind of deodorant does Batman use?"

Apparently Batman does not use Degree deodorant.

"Right Guard!" I reply with confidence.

"Yeah," he agrees. "Batman uses Right Guard."

"Daddy," Cade's trivia ensues. "What kind of deodorant does The Flash use?"

Over the course of the next fifteen minutes I learn the deodorant choices of each member of the Justice League team. I stand by watching Cade as he adds a sixth container of deodorant to our shopping cart. His pursuit of antiperspirant knowledge slows and I notice a discomfort that's building in his eyes. It's evident that a migraine is on the way. Grabbing Excedrin from the nearby aisle, I hand Cade my shaken iced tea that I just purchased from the instore Starbucks shop. Quietly we sit on the industrial tiled floor. I've come to dread moments like this. It's always nerve wrecking knowing that at any moment the two of us could be wrestling across the store's Metamucil display.

"Stop at Target on the way home." I text to Julee. "I just gave Cade some Excedrin and we are doing fine right now."

"Living now," she replies.

"Living now," is the message that she sends me every day as she heads home from work.

"Dad," Cade looks at me glossy eyed. "Don't make the Hulk angry. He would not be..."

Cade waits for me to complete his sentence. I know exactly the word he expects from me but I refuse to give in.

"He would not be pleased," I suggest.

"Dad," again he looks over. "Don't make the Hulk angry. He would not be…"

"He would not be thrilled about it."

I continue my refusal to give in. I refuse to give in to the "H" word. Although it may seem silly, I know that if I say "happy," Cade will start to scream. It's just one of the things that he does when he's upset.

"Dad," he attempts once more. "Don't make the Hulk angry. He would not be…"

"The hulk would not be delighted."

Slowly Cade's eyes close as he leans back against the shelf. I pull the deodorant from our cart and smile at the toddler passing by. The young boy drools and then smiles back at us. His long sandy blonde hair is stuck to the saliva on his chubby pink cheeks. Looking down he reaches into his bag of strawberry Twizzlers. In an unselfish gesture he offers one to Cade.

"Thank you," I acknowledge the boy's kindness.

Gently, his mother grabs his hand and together they move on. Holding his candy twist, Cade leans just slightly forward.

"Daddy," he grins. "Twizzlers makes your mouth…"

"Twizzlers makes your mouth happy!" And just like that, Daddy gets tricked.

"He is not HAP-PY! He is not HAP-PY!"

Each repeated phrase gets progressively louder. He snaps his string of licorice onto the floor.

"He is not HAP-PY! He is not HAP-PY!"

Cade slams his head vigorously against the rows of deodorant. Degree hits the floor. Mitchum hits the floor. Right Guard hits the floor. Old Spice goes flying. With a tube of Mennen Speed Stick in my hand I call for Cade's attention.

"I'm General Zod." In a puppet-like manner, I manipulate the container's cap. "Have you seen Superman?"

A confused Cade looks me over from head to toe. Wrinkling his forehead, he glances at the Speed Stick that's in my hand. Dropping his shredded candy remnants, he grabs a tube of Degree deodorant.

"You'll never get away with this Zod!" He declares.

There's an epic battle of good vs evil, Speed Stick vs Degree, taking place on aisle five. I never knew that antiperspirant could be so much fun. All is calm by the time Julee arrives. We restock the shelves and head back to the house. Somehow, we managed to find the ingredients for my grandmother's cobbler recipe. Everything but those wondrous dark purple mulberries, that is. Looks like we'll be having blackberry cobbler instead.

We get home and Julee applies cream to the scratches on my arm. "Here Baby… Try this. It will help keep you from scarring."

We sit at the table as Cade plays with his action figures.

"Some women would consider it strange finding their husband playing with deodorant in the supermarket." Grabbing my hand Julee looks towards me. "I feel sorry for them. They're missing out on a really good thing."

Don't Squeeze the Spaceman's Taco

I preheat the oven to 350 degrees and then join Cade on the living room floor. Taking a deep breath, Julee lifts the bag of store bought ingredients. She inserts the movie *Chocolat* into our portable DVD player and then kicks her shoes to the side. As Cade and I play with his DC collectibles, Julee blends the ingredients to the beat of the movie's classic score. With her mixer set to medium speed, she whisks the sugar, flour, milk and melted butter. Slowly she pours the batter into a greased baking dish while her hips continue to sway. Lovingly, she adds a layer of frozen Target berries. It's not exactly my grandmother's cobbler. But frozen berries, love and a sprinkle of sugar and you're bound to make something worthwhile.

The movie continues playing. *Chocolat* is one of Julee's favorites. She watches the film every Good Friday in the morning just before heading to cousin Pat's for the annual rolling of the "cock."

Golden brown and bubbling, an hour later the cobbler is ready. Cade and I are still playing in the living room. Carrying one of our blue glazed pottery bowls in each hand, Julee approaches. The bowls are filled with fresh baked cobbler and scoops of vanilla ice cream melting on top.

"I didn't see the condensed milk in the bag," she tells me.

"I must have forgotten to pick it up," I reply sliding the empty can quietly under the couch.

Cade and I finished the entire can; one spoonful at a time while playing superheroes on the living room floor.

As usual, it takes a heap of energy to clean the mess that's left in our kitchen. Julee cooks and I do the cleaning. That's how it works at our house. As I scrub the baking dish, Julee emerges from the hall bathroom. In her hand she's holding the Gillette Venus that she uses to shave her legs. Puzzled, she stares at the wiry bouquet of pubic hairs attached to its blade.

"A hoo-ha razor!" I yell in excitement. "I finally know what a hoo-ha razor is."

Every parent is going to have to deal with sexuality at some point and it's best to be proactive. Although Cade is innocent in many ways, he's still a teenage boy. This is evident by his bashful looks while online looking at pictures of Selena Gomez.

Growing up, I learned many things about sex from my peers. I realize that Cade doesn't have the same opportunity. Therefore, I do what I can to be his best friend as well as his dad. Having a hoo-ha can be complicated. If I can teach him appropriateness and safety when it comes to his hoo-ha, then I consider that a job well done.

Chapter 6

Roar

Weekend mornings I look forward to sleeping late. I don't know why because it never seems to happen. It's a Sunday morning and I could really use some extra snooze time. In need of inspiration, I stayed up past 2:00 a.m. chatting with my mom.

"Why is the neighbor running a chainsaw so early in the morning?" Julee moans while elbowing me on my side.

"How the hell am I supposed to know?"

"Would you go check?"

"Why do I need to go check?"

"Please," she begs. "If it's Jennifer, tell her that we'll go help her out later if she doesn't mind stopping."

"Okay! Okay! I'll go check."

Rolling out of bed I notice the time.

"Who the fuck runs a chainsaw at 6:00 a.m.?" I ramble while stumbling down the hallway.

Still half asleep I open the front door. Nothing unusual other than the stray cat staring back at me -- Mr. Yang we call him.

"I don't have anything for you, Yang." I tell him.

For some reason Mr. Yang doesn't believe me and he moves in a little closer. Squatting on the front step, I lower my hand. We sit there a bit, Yang and I, as he brushes his head along my fingertips. What a quiet and peaceful morning. Quiet and peaceful outside, that is. The thundering commotion was actually coming from indoors, Brett's bedroom to be exact. It turns out that the chainsaw we heard was just Brett singing "Walking on Sunshine" by Katrina and the Waves. Knocking on Brett's bedroom door, I ask if he'd postpone his concert until after 9:00 a.m.

"Why," he questions. "Was I being loud?"

"It's not me Brett," I assure him. "I love your singing. It's your sister. She thought that you were a chainsaw."

"Really?" He asks.

"Really." I reply.

"Well that's OK." Brett tells me. "I'm not mad."

When Brett says, "I'm not mad." It means only one thing. He's mad. Anytime Brett is mad or remotely nervous, he does his best to change the subject.

Pacing the floor in front of his Sony PlayStation, he rolls the left sleeve of his Five Finger Death Punch tee shirt up to his shoulder. His Tootsie Roll pajama pants are pulled nipple high.

"Look Kell...I was watching *Law and Order* and there was an asshole that beat up his girlfriend. And you know what?"

"What Brett?"

"They killed that son of a bitch and you know what else?"

"What's that?"

"He deserved it." Still distraught about cancelling his morning concert he continues. "You still gonna take me for a driving lesson?"

Brett's biggest dream is to one day have a vehicle of his own. He's attempted the driving test on numerous occasions but has failed each time. Periodically I let him drive my car on vacant streets and empty parking lots. I do this at late hours when there are no other cars around, or people, or mailboxes, or homes for that matter -- nothing that he could possibly run into.

"Brett," I remember shouting as he hopped the curb. "Would you please get the car off the sidewalk?"

Although skillful with video games, he's something else behind the wheel.

"Trust me Kell." He replied while continuing his drive along the sidewalk. "I have lots of patience…You know that? I am very patient."

When Brett says that he has patience, it means only one thing. He's losing his patience.

"Yes Brett," I assured him. "You are very patient. Now would you patiently get the car off the sidewalk and get back onto the street?"

Thinking about my previous driving lessons with Brett, I roll my eyes. "Of course I'll take you for a driving lesson."

"Oh goodie." He replies.

Grabbing his TV remote, his nervous pacing comes to an end. He lets out a sigh of relief and sits back comfortably on his reclining leather chair.

"I'm sorry for waking up my sister." He continues. "I'll sing later because that's what gangstas do."

"Thank you Brett. You're right. That is what gangstas do." Pointing towards him I reassure. "And you are definitely a gangsta."

I step over Gumbo who's lying quietly on the floor beside Brett's bed and I close the door. Feeling a bit thirsty, I head to the kitchen for a glass of water. I always enjoy a squeeze of lemon in my water so I open the refrigerator.

No matter how many times I see this, it always cracks me up. On any given day Brett leaves a large can of cheap beer in the fridge. Now this may not seem odd at first, but picture this:

- The can is usually half empty with a paper towel shoved into the opening to preserve its freshness. Brett finishes the rest of the beer over the course of the next day or two. The idea of day old cheap beer that has gone flat does absolutely nothing for me. However, I applaud Brett for his resourcefulness.

"Now that's gangsta!" Thinking out loud I close the fridge.

With a song in my head, I walk on sunshine back to my bedroom. Brett's concert is to continue in less than three hours and I really need some rest. Still beaming I crawl into bed.

"Thank you for doing that." Julee mutters. "Was everything all right?"

"Yes." I tell her as I tug firmly on our quilt. "Jennifer said that she would wait until after 9:00 a.m. before she cranks up the chainsaw again."

I look over to check the time on my phone and notice Mom's message.

"His Everlasting Friendship"

The midst of loneliness is gone
The light of love is here
Come share the boundless friendship
He's ruling everywhere
Come hear the voice of gladness
Give thankfulness each day
The angel of the Lord has come
To give and show the way
I feel a great tomorrow
It's living in my soul
Come to the banquet supper
His love is from of old
He's master of his handiwork
Creation comes alive
He's greater than the universe
He's ever at my side
A time of great rejoicing
Redeeming grace for all
He's given us a miracle
We listen to the call

Helen Melerine

"I love you Mom." Closing my eyes, I drift back to sleep.

Moments later my eyes are wide open. It's exactly 9:00 am and three hours have literally passed in the blink of an eye. Ironically, I'm awakened by Metallica's "Enter Sandman." And Julee was right. It really does sound like a chainsaw.

I walk into the kitchen with my Earbuds shoved tightly into my ear canals. There's no drowning out the clamor that's coming from Brett's bedroom. Clearing my throat, I answer my phone.

"Hello Nana."

It's my sister Iris. Cade calls her Nana and so I answer her calls, "Hello Nana."

"I'm sorry. Did I wake you?" She asks.

"No," regretfully I reply. "I'm up."

"Oh, I woke you up. Go back to sleep."

"No, seriously." I reiterate.

To prove that she didn't wake me up, I slide my phone under Brett's door. Immediately, she bursts into laughter.

"You did not wake me up."

Still laughing she replies. "I forgot why I called…Yeah, now I remember. I found Cade's old otoscope."

"Wow! I remember those days."

There was a time when Cade put everything imaginable into his ears. This we called the squirreling phase. Like a squirrel harvesting nuts for winter, Cade transformed his boring hollow ear canals into caverns of hidden treasures. It was discovered one day when we noticed him pulling on his ear lobes and screaming. There was a stomach churning odor coming from his ears like a milkshake left in a parked car -- outside in the summer sun – for somewhere between a week or two. With what seemed like an infection, we took Cade to our family doctor. He was prescribed antibiotics as well as ibuprofen for inflammation.

A couple days later, I noticed Cade biting his fingernails and squirreling them away. Holding the jagged tip of his pinky fingernail out in front of him, he admired it one last time. Then, with his head bent low to the ground, he buried it deep within his auricle. My initial thought was that these fingernail pieces may have reached his ear drum causing pain and infection.

With his otoscope in hand the doctor carefully searched.

"I don't see anything," he announced.

Looking a second time, he tugged at Cade's ear.

"Wait a minute."

"Do you see a fingernail?" I asked.

"No." The doctor replied. "It looks like a tiny plastic ball or pellet of some sort. But it's really close to his ear drum."

Not wanting to harm Cade's ears, he referred us to an Ear, Nose and Throat specialist. The ENT noticed the plastic ball as well as another tiny rock. He attempted to remove the items while we were in his office, but Cade refused to sit still. The objects that Cade hoarded into his ear canals were now driving him nuts Therefore, we had no other choice but to schedule an outpatient procedure.

Nervously, Julee and I sat in the waiting room of the local hospital. Cade was sedated and the doctor performed the task at hand.

The clock ticked loudly.

It was a quick procedure. However, if you asked us it felt like an eternity. And within ten minutes of starting, the doctor was finished.

"I examined both ears thoroughly and everything has been removed." The doctor informed us while holding a plastic prescription bottle in his hand. "Never have I seen such a unique assortment of objects in one patient's ears." Smiling, he handed us the bottle. "Cade is quite the collector."

Curiously, I unscrewed the bottle's cap. Within it there were treasures untold.

- one small plastic pellet
- six tiny rocks
- four jagged fingernails
- one half inch piece of plastic from Julee's hair clip
- one Shrek colored crayon tip (a murky pea green – the color of his favorite Ogre)
- and three grains of Uncle Ben's instant brown rice

Following the procedure Cade was calm and relaxed. With his ears free of all debris, I knew that my son had finally learned his lesson.

Wrong!

Before long we were back at the hospital removing the new treasures that he squirreled away. After Cade's second outpatient procedure we decided to purchase our own otoscope. Several times per day we examined his ears. Anything new was immediately flushed with water. Cade's squirreling phase went on for quite some time. Continuously, he placed items into his ears. And continuously he panicked when he couldn't get them out. Although we were able to remove most items at home, there were some that still required a doctor's visit. However, Cade was no longer the frightened little boy that wouldn't sit still. He now knew exactly what to expect and sat giggling while the doctor did his job.

The following summer, Cade spent a couple months with his Nana. In addition to his usual belongings, we also packed an otoscope and syringe for flushing. My sister is very attentive with Cade. One day while playing outside she noticed that Cade was tugging at his ear. Holding the otoscope tightly in her hand, she carefully searched.

"What's that?" She thought as she continued observing.

"Cade," she asked. "Did you put something in your ear?"

Before Cade could answer she noticed the tiny legs moving.

"A bug!" He proudly exclaimed.

Within moments they were at the doctor's office and the bug was killed with a few drops of mineral oil. Upon removal of the dead bug, the doctor informed my sister that insects don't always back up. I envisioned a picture of Cade's ear on the cover of an old Roach Motel box. "Roaches check in, but they don't check out!"

As I'm talking to my sister, I can feel cracked fragments of glass scraping against my cheek. The sharp edges remind me of Cade's latest phase.

"He's now searching images on electronic devices and smacking them." I tell her. "I'm constantly yelling, 'Cade, don't hit your tablet!' or 'Cade, don't hit my phone!' or 'Cade, don't hit the computer!'"

"Does he stop?" She asks.

"Briefly," I reply. "But only to laugh and say, 'It's not nice to hit Atticus Finch.' Exactly how am I supposed to respond to that?"

When Cade is feeling good he finds it hilarious to hit images of the character Atticus Finch from *To Kill a Mockingbird*. However, when he's hurting he searches for images of other things -- things that piss him off. They're just odd images. Why they piss him off? I have no idea. But he searches for these random images and then hits the screen hard enough to shatter the glass. As a result, I've gotten to know the electronic repairman quite well.

"It's just a phase," I tell myself.

Like his many other phases I anxiously await this one ending. It's becoming rather expensive.

"It will pass." Iris assures me. "Remember when everything started with 'E'?"

"God yes," I tell her. "How can I forget? I have no idea why he insisted that all words start with the letter 'E.' He's actually quite good at spelling. One time we were at a restaurant and I asked Cade to order from the menu. He started by saying, 'Hamburger please.' I was really proud of him. He ordered exactly what he wanted and he even said please"

"What happened next?" Iris asks.

"Well, next the server asked if he would like fries and Cade responded, 'Fries starts with 'E.'" The server then played along and said, 'No, fries starts with 'F.'"

"That's cute."

"That's cute until ten minutes later Cade has recited all of the menu items that start with the letter 'E.' Which, by the way, happened to be the entire menu."

Iris was in the delivery room when Cade was born and she has been with us through every one of his many challenging phases.

"Aww, remember when he used to bite the DVD's?" She asks.

"Oh yeah… I remember that. 'You can't eat DVD's. They are not food. They are not delicious.' I remember that very well actually. Thank God for video streaming. Our DVD collection now looks like leftovers from a Golden Corral buffet."

It feels good to laugh at these things that used to frustrate me. From flushing toys down the toilet to questioning everyone about their appliance ownership, the madness can be downright hilarious at times.

"What kind of stove do you have?"

"What kind of dishwasher do you have?"

"What kind of refrigerator do you have?"

"What kind of toaster do you have?"

"What kind of cutter plugger do you have?"

A cutter plugger, by the way, is what Cade calls an electric can opener. Talking to Iris I failed to notice that the noise from Brett's room has already come to an end. I step into the family room and something beautiful catches my eye.

The hummingbird feeder dangles near our picture window. From inside I watch the marvel of the tiny creature. Heavy footsteps quickly approach from outside and away scatters the little bird. Brother-in-law Brett swiftly runs by. His pudgy belly leads the way to the shed behind our house.

"Brum…..brum……brum."

Brett cranks his scooter. I wait at the window and watch as he zips on by. His helmet is fastened tightly above his head. A smile is stretched happily across his face. The little scooter provides Brett with an immense amount of freedom. We have learned that it's best to have two scooters. This way when one is inevitably in need of repair, the other one is ready on standby. We've also learned not to park our vehicles anywhere near the shed.

"Hey…um…Darrin!" exclaimed Brett to my nephew Darrin who was visiting us. "You need to move your car. I keep running into it."

The day that Brett gets a driver's license I will alert everyone to stay indoors. Until then he's hell on wheels with 50 cubic centimeters of power or less.

    Brett loves the independence that owning a scooter has given him. He has become quite an avid local traveler. Constantly, I give him talks on the importance of safety. And although Brett takes his scooter safety very serious, I remain worried. My worries are especially heightened in periods of inclement weather. Regardless of my worries, Brett insists on riding his scooter come rain or come shine. However, there is one thing that will always stop him in his tracks and that's lightning. He is terribly afraid of lightning.

One evening while attending a wedding a little over ninety miles away in the mountains, I received a call from Brett.

    "Um…Kelly," he uttered. "I'm going home from the book store and I just saw lightning."

    "Where are you?" I asked.

    "I am on the side of the road waiting."

    "What are you waiting for?" I asked.

"I am waiting for the lightning to stop. I don't want to be struck by lightning."

"Is it raining heavily?" I continued.

"Well...um...It hasn't started raining yet." He replied.

"How far are you from the house?"

"I'm a little pass Burger King."

"Well Brett, that's only two miles from the house. So your best bet is to get on your scooter and get your ass home before the rain…"

Immediately I'm interrupted, "I don't want to get struck by lightning!"

With my fingers tightly crossed, I promised Brett that he wouldn't be struck by lightning that evening. Lightning is the only naturally occurring phenomenon that will keep him off of his scooter. I am always offering Brett transportation to wherever he wishes to go. But, the only way that he accepts my offer is if both scooters have malfunctioned. There once was a time when one of his scooters was in the shop getting repaired and the other one had a faulty headlight. We informed Brett that he should only use his scooter to go short distances and only during daylight hours. Nonetheless, Brett decided that it was a good idea to go to the movie theater. Although there was daylight when the movie started, there was none when the movie ended. Julee received that call.

"Um…Julee," he stuttered. "You need to come and get me. I am at the movies and my headlight isn't working."

Julee approached Brett at the curb in front of the box office ticket booth and he entered her vehicle. She let him know that I would be back to retrieve his scooter later with my trailer. Upon exiting the parking lot Brett asked Julee to stop and back up.

"I forgot something in my scooter," he stated.

"What is it?" She asked.

"Um…I forgot my beer."

"Your beer? What the hell are you doing with beer on your scooter?"

Brett pointed to the spot where his scooter was parked. It was the space closest to the theater entrance. With a locking cable intact, it was securely fastened to the adjacent sign which read "Police Vehicle Parking Only." Julee's stern advice instructed Brett to move his scooter to a new location. With his locking cable in hand he searched for the next best thing -- a handicap sign. Content with his new parking spot, he grabbed his beer and reentered Julee's vehicle. The look on her face told him to get out and try again.

"That's OK," Brett responded. "I'm not mad. I'll just look for a better place to park."

At the far end of the lot stood a row of blooming Crepe Myrtles, a staple among southern landscapes. With their bright red summer flowers and smooth surface barks, it was undoubtedly a lovely place to secure his beloved scooter. Satisfied with Brett's new parking choice they both drove back to the house. Julee was relieved to discover that the beer had not been opened. His true intention was to savor his Pabst Blue Ribbon at home over the next couple days. As we've come to learn from

Brett, a tall can of cheap beer and a torn paper towel means the party never ends.

Meanwhile, I returned home from the nearby Lowe's. I had just purchased a bottle of nectar for our hummingbird feeder and a few solar landscaping lights for our garden. It was once again time to replace the lights at the front corner of the house. They were really easy to install. I just attached them to their accompanying spikes and into the ground they went.

As Julee drove by she rolled down her window.

"Boy do I have a story to tell you." She sighed.

She parked her vehicle behind our house; far away from the shed of course. Rapid stomping approached and brother-in-law Brett jogged hurriedly by. As he made that dreaded right turn I could hear him shout.

"I didn't do it!"

And that was the last time that I replaced our landscaping lights. Smiling from my memories of that crazy day, I walk outside. Jennifer is busy trimming the shrubbery surrounding her house. With a tight grip on her pruning shears, she clips away. I shake my head as I envision a roaring chainsaw within her grasp. Slowly my eyes drift downward and to my surprise, our landscaping lights are still intact. Our nearby gardenias; however, didn't fare so well. With their dry brown leaves, I know right away that they had fallen victim to the wrath of Brett's Reeboks.

I walk back into the house and without Brett's singing, our home is unusually quiet. A faint noise echoes from the bathroom and I stroll down the hallway to investigate the sound.

"Gillette," Cade stares into the mirror. "The best a man can get."

With one eyebrow raised, his electric razor buzzes as he prepares for a shave.

Reluctantly, my laughter gives me away.

"Dad," he asks. "What kind of razor does Austin Powers use?"

"I don't know," I reply. "What kind of razor does he use?"

"He uses Gillette," Cade informs me. Then, in in his best Austin Powers voice, Cade continues, "Yeah baby! Yeah!"

Smiling, I watch Cade stroke his face.

"Very shagadelic!" He proudly exclaims.

"Yes Cade." I agree. "Very shagadelic indeed."

Pleased with Cade's interest in grooming, I head back to the kitchen. I pick up his dirty socks off of the floor and throw them into our hamper.

"Coffee…coffee…coffee…"

In a zombie-like trance Julee enters the room.

"Good morning." Yawning, she leans her head against my back.

"Good morning." I turn around to give her a hug.

"Thank you for making coffee."

"You bet. Did you get enough sleep?"

"No," she continues. "But I was too tired to get out of bed."

Steam rises as she pours her cup. Growing up along the bayou, we like our coffee strong. Julee sighs and inhales the dark aromatic blend.

"Remember Maw-Maw Tonia's coffee?" With her eyes closed, Julee inhales once more.

Maw-Maw Tonia was my paternal grandmother. She was a descendant of the Canary Islands. Los Islenos, they were called, a group of islanders that settled in St. Bernard Parish in the late 1700's. She spoke an outdated Spanish which was actually more of an outdated Spanglish. Whenever my grandmother and I talked, I usually found myself lost somewhere mid-sentence. Regretfully, my generation was the first to not learn the native Islenos language. Maw-Maw Tonia was a hard-working woman that maintained her rich Canarian heritage. Her coffee; however, was undeniably New Orleans.

"I sure do miss her café au lait." Thinking of my mornings with my grandmother I continue. "She definitely gave Café du Monde a run for their money."

For over two hundred years, New Orleanians have made their morning Joe with boiled milk and dark black coffee & chicory. In spite of all that, there was something uniquely different about the way my grandmother prepared hers. Of course, no one ever found out. Although Maw-Maw Tonia freely gave out her most prized recipes, there was always a missing ingredient. This insured her the upper hand. Some may call that cheating, but she called it winning. Just ask the ladies that played Pitty Pat with her on any given Saturday night. They'd tell you that Maw-Maw Tonia always won. Now I'm not saying that she cheated, but you can bet that there was always a couple extra aces that she kept hidden deep within the back pockets of her polyester slacks.

Savoring her cup of coffee, Julee softly grabs my hand and leads me to the living room. "Come watch the Food Network with me."

Julee loves watching the Food Network. "It's therapeutic," she says. Following her footsteps, I join her in front of the television for a little couple's therapy. Five minutes later I'm surfing the web on my cell phone.

"Why don't you put down your phone and watch this with me?"

"I'm watching," I insist.

"Uh-huh," sarcastically she agrees. "You're doing what you always do. You're playing on your phone."

"I am not. Now you know there's nothing I enjoy more than spending time with you, Paula Dean and a stick of butter."

"Uh-huh," she lovingly pokes me on the side.

Couple's therapy is shortly lived as Cade enters the room.

"Daddy," Cade shouts as he joins us on the couch. "Who's Dora like from *Dora the Explorer?*"

When Cade is present, he takes center stage.

"Dora is like Ms. Leidy," I reply.

"Yeah," he agrees and smiles. "Daddy, who's Diego like from *Go Diego, Go*?"

"Diego is like Mr. Carlos."

"Yeah." Loudly, he asks another question. "Daddy, who would make a good Wonder Woman for Halloween."

"Nelly Furtado."

"Daddy..." with a high pitch he squeals, "Shrek!"

"Shrek!" I squeal back at him.

Distracted from her cooking show Julee asks, "Cade, what would you like for lunch today?"

"Food." He quickly responds.

"What kind of food?"

"What kind of food?" He repeats the question. "Let's see...umm...How about Mediterranean food?"

"That sounds good, Cade." Julee continues. "Who eats Mediterranean food?"

"Aladdin!"

"That's right baby...Aladdin. I'm going to finish watching my show and then I'll get started on lunch." Eager to learn the final steps of Paula Dean's shrimp and rice dish, Julee waits. "Oh no, Cade! You changed the channel."

Good-bye Paula Dean. Hello *Teen Titans*. Inspired by the Food Network, Julee works like a maniac all afternoon in the kitchen -- chopping onions, grinding chickpeas, mixing sauces and cleaning the good China.

"We're having kibbeh and stuffed grape leaves for lunch. Would you grab another jar of grape leaves from the cabinet?"

She asks. "I have enough ingredients to make extra and I'd like to send some to Aunt Delores."

Reaching for the jar, I'm reminded of the day that we purchased the grape leaves from the supermarket. It all started with our barking dogs.

"Ruff ruff…woof woof…ruff ruff…woof… " Tramp and Gumbo jumped at the door awaiting the person on the other side. "Woof woof…ruff…"

"Shut up!" I shouted. "It's just Brett coming home from the gym."

"Oh, hey Gumbo" Brett announced as he entered the doorway. "Hey Tramp. How are you today?"

"I'm fine. Now get out of my fucking way." Brett mumbled in his best Tramp voice.

"Man you hear that dog?" Brett exclaimed. "He told me to get out of his way."

It may seem a bit odd that my brother-in-law speaks to the dogs. However, it"s even more odd that they speak back to him. Exactly what are the dogs trying to convey through their barking? And why do I fuss at them when they bark? Am I just being a jerk?

Tramp: "Wow! I love your new shoes. Those wingtips are really flattering on you."

Me: "Piss off you stupid dog. Now go lay down and be quiet."

I think Brett has it right. However, I can't help but find myself yelling at the dogs every time that they start barking. Why should I yell? I know that dogs bark. I knew that before I had them. I also know that cows moo, pigs oink and lions roar. I don't own any of those, by the way.

"See you later Brett." Heading out the door to go grocery shopping, we bid each other farewell.

"See you later Tote!" Brett quickly replied.

"Yeah, see you later," grumbling in his Tramp voice he added. "You fucking tote."

It was a busy weekend morning at the local supermarket. Julee thoroughly scanned the aisle for a jar of grape leaves. Holding her family's Lebanese cookbook, Julee scanned, I stood by and Cade stimmed.

When Cade is experiencing anxiety or stress he may start flapping his hands and repeating phrases. Therapists call this self-stimulatory behavior or stimming. It's a coping mechanism that helps him to remain calm. To be honest, I didn't know what to think when I first noticed this behavior myself. My instinct was to tell him to stop. After all, I didn't want him to look "odd" in public. I soon realized why he did it and from that moment on, I welcomed it.

A pudgy man who appeared to be in his mid-thirties entered from the far end of the aisle. Following behind were his two young daughters. The girls both had long dirty blonde hair that bounced as they walked a happy step. Their beautiful smiles and matching Hannah Montana t-shirts caused me to smile in return. As they approached I noticed the gentleman staring at Cade's stimming. Walking by, I heard him mutter, "That kid's an idiot."

Pausing in disbelief, I asked myself, "Did I just hear him correctly?"

"He doesn't know any better." I tried to rationalize with myself.

"Why would a grown man say something like this to his children?" I just didn't understand.

"Why would a grown man say something like this about my child?"

Furiously, I pushed my shopping cart aside. Kicking off my flip flops, I ran after the tubby bastard. With my blood pressure rising, I clenched him by the collar. I don't remember the exact words used but I laid into that piece of shit. It took everything in me not to smash his face into the adjacent cans of okra.

An image of Miley Cyrus popped into my head and I suddenly remembered his children. Pushing the man aside I shouted, "Go team Miley!"

It was a great lecture I gave at the supermarket that day. I taught some idiot that it's okay for a person to stim. Some may call that revenge. I call it autism awareness. I also learned a couple of lessons myself. I learned that despite all the unwanted noise, it's okay for a dog to bark. I owe Tramp and Gumbo an apology for that. More importantly, I also learned that just like a cow moos and just like a pig oinks; if someone messes with your kid, then you better believe that it's okay for a lion to roar.

P.S. Please don't ask me what happened at Chuck E Cheese's.

Chapter 7

Finding Respite

What is beauty? Sometime it's evident in obvious physical characteristics. Sometime it's right in front of you and sometime you have to search. Sometime it's beautiful from the beginning and sometime what starts out ugly turns into something beautiful.

Amid the tall palm trees and cerulean Atlantic shore, Castaway Cay would be a great place to spend an eternity. At least Julee thinks so. This is where she would like her remains to be spread one day. The 1,000 acre paradise serves as an exclusive port for the Disney Cruise Line. I just hope the lush bougainvillea and Bahamian calypso tunes create a big enough distraction. My plan is to carry her ashes in a tequila bottle. She prefers Jose Cuervo. As I bask in the warm tropical sun, I will say good-bye one margarita glass at a time. Cade was only three years old on our first visit to this private oasis. It was then that Julee fell in love with the place.

There is beauty in the world. What an amazing creator we must have to spawn such splendor. Julee, on the other hand, is far more beautiful than all thousand acres combined. She doubts herself at times. However, that's one of the things that makes her so beautiful. Her love and support for me make her even more beautiful. I could go on and on but at some point it would just get sickening. There's one aspect of her beauty, however, I just can't ignore. The love and sacrifice involved with raising my son is worthy of a monument rivaling the Taj Mahal. Unfortunately, I am not so wealthy and I would have to construct such a monument from clearance items bought at the local Hobby Lobby.

There is beauty in the world. Raising a child with disabilities is grueling. It's easy to be overwhelmed with grief when thinking of the life that could have been. However, it's beautiful appreciating the life that is. Sometime we don't appreciate our own beautiful lives until we realize how screwed up life is for others. Some people call this, "counting your blessings." I call it, "not counting your troubles." It's the only thing keeping me from being a raging alcoholic.

Most mornings with Cade are challenging. It's not uncommon for me to look like a cage fighter by the time breakfast is over. The key word there is "over." When it's over, it's time to move on. There is no time for grudges. On the other hand, there is plenty time for forgiveness. Forgiveness gives me the opportunity to enjoy the many beautiful moments shared with my son. Forgiveness is a true thing of beauty. Forgiveness gives me the strength to appreciate days like today.

Cade and I sit down for breakfast. Close your eyes and imagine a dimly lit brunch; the type you find at an elegant five star resort. Now open them and find two bowls of Captain America cereal and an IPad playing random nonsense Cade found on YouTube. In case you're curious, Captain America cereal is kind of like re-shaped Alpha Bits cereal with marshmallows resembling Captain America's shield. Nonetheless, it's quality time.

Allergies in the Carolinas are a bitch. Before long I started sneezing. Sneezing always makes me nervous. Why? Because I know that if I am sneezing Cade may soon be sneezing as well. The problem being that allergies trigger Cade's migraines. Our giggling father and son time ends with a torn shirt, cracked door, broken lamp, scratched arms and Captain America marshmallows shoved up my nose. What a crappy way to start the day. In fact it's down-right ugly. However, that doesn't mean it has to end that way.

I send Julee out for some retail therapy. It would have been nice to spend Mother's Day together but in our house you learn to go with the flow. Gone was my vision of Ward and June on a Sunday stroll with the Beaver. Today my Beaver was more like the pissed off dog in Stephen King's *Cujo*. I kiss Julee good-bye and re-enter the boxing ring.

A couple hours later a friend messages me asking about my day. This is my reply:

"Good. But then again my definition of good most would call chaos. My son had a migraine and took it out on the furniture and on my arms. However, once his firestorm was over, the two of us hung out, watched 007 kick ass on Netflix and ate Chinese take-out."

Today, what started out ugly turned into something beautiful. If you ask me, James Bond and Chinese food go together like red beans and rice. Cade and I enjoy an eight hour action movie marathon before Julee returns home.

"Thanks for sending me out. I really needed it." Relaxed, yet worn out from her day of shopping, she sits beside us. "Wait until you see the great deals that I found."

The number of bags on the floor let me know that I would regret the upcoming credit card statement. Nonetheless, it's cheaper than a therapist. Dealing with the terrible two's is trying for most parents. Julee and I have been dealing with the terrible two's for over fifteen years. When caring for a disabled loved one it's easy to become stressed out and exhausted. It's easy to become so wrapped up in taking care of them that we forget to take care of ourselves.

Finding respite is an important part of the caregiving process. With no relief from the madness, a breakdown would be inevitable. Respite care can be found through many service care providers. It can also be found through the help of true friends and family. Julee and I most often rely upon each other.

Many times we feel guilty at the thought of needing relief. What kind of parent needs relief from their child? Truth being a little break always did wonders for Cade and for us as well. Upon leaving my job to stay home with Cade, I lost track of who I was as a person. I knew that I was a father. That part remained constant. Nonetheless, there was still something that was missing.

I'm six months into being a stay at home dad and it's turning out to be just another typical mid-week day. Between making breakfast, taking Cade to school, changing the sheets, watching my stock symbols and cleaning Brett's damned toilet, the spinning wheel is beginning to make me dizzy. I log off my stock trading account and log into Facebook instead. Through social media I enjoy the usual political bickering, the usual Jesus loves me and hates you and the usual selfie-stick overkill. Scrolling through my timeline, a random posting catches my eye. Charlotte International Fashion Week is holding a model call for their upcoming event.

I did the whole modeling thing back in the early nineties. Back then I was represented by the same talent agent as Britney Spears. At the time, Britney was still an unknown young dreamer living in Kentwood, Louisiana. Karen Berthelot, owner of Glamour Modeling; however, saw something bigger in Britney. It was something that the rest of the world would soon discover as well. Although I lacked the drive that Britney had, Karen was a big influence in my life. Her guidance has helped me to overcome many obstacles ever since. It's amazing how simple lessons can become lifelong principles.

Don't Squeeze the Spaceman's Taco

It was the summer of 1992, just four months after Julee and I tied the knot. An offer was presented by a top agent to go test shooting in Milan, Italy. Rather than go to Milan, I decided to work longer hours instead. My goal was to save money, pay down bills and then pursue my dreams.

Over twenty years have passed since then. Regrettably, I still haven't saved money, I still have bills, and somewhere on the backburner I still have dreams. I attend the casting call. In my mid-forties, I'm twice the age of almost everyone else there. Two days later I receive a call informing me that I have been selected. I know nothing of the underground fashion scene in Charlotte, NC. I've never seen so many beautiful people with radiant, flawless skin in one room before. I had no idea that local designers are fetching more for their outfits than I'm paying for my mortgage. To me, modeling is just an escape. It's a way of having a life outside of being a caregiver. With the connections that I make, my modeling hobby lands me in cities throughout the country. The best part is that I'm able make some great new friends. Friends that I encourage to dream. Friends that go on to successful careers in the industry. Watching these young people succeed brings me great joy. Being a "responsible" dreamer my whole life, I encourage them to do otherwise.

The fashion seen gives me and Julee a much needed break. But that's pretty much all that I consider it—a break. My passion, my goals, my dreams all revolve around my son. With every breath that I take, I think of him. Knowing that he will never be independent weighs heavily on my soul. Every time that I cook a meal he enjoys, I'm left to wonder, "Who will do this when I am gone?" Every time that I take him to the movies or the amusement park, I wonder, "Who will do this when I am gone?" Who's going to take care of my buddy when I am gone?

Just like the young dreamers that I've met in the fashion industry, I know that Cade has dreams. I just have no idea what they are. Everyone has dreams. I often wonder as I stroll the city streets, "What was his dream?" Growing up, I don't recall any kids in my neighborhood dreaming of being bankers or cab drivers. Nonetheless, there certainly are plenty of bankers and cab drivers out there. I don't recall any kids dreaming of being janitors or accountants neither. Yet janitors and accountants are a dime a dozen. And never do I recall anyone ever dreaming of being homeless. Unfortunately, homelessness is a reality for far too many. When did the dream die? Dreams are like a fire. They require kindling.

What is Cade's dream? I would give anything to find out. When I tell him to blow out his candles and make a wish, does he even know what a wish is? For Cade's last birthday we had those annoying reigniting candles. Just like dreams, some flames ceased and some came back stronger. Some flames weakened and some were replaced by others.

Granted I may never know Cade's true wishes, but I do know mine. It's funny how they can change over time. While I once dreamed that Cade would be the rock star / astronaut that I never was, I now cling to the hope that he will never be homeless. We're all similar creatures. Our prayers and wishes change according to our own level of desperation.

"Dear God, please help me to get this promotion so that I can buy that beautiful new house by the lake."

"Dear God, please help me to keep the lights on and to keep food on the table."

"Dear God, I've been constipated for weeks. Please help me to have just one good bowel movement."

My advice to the youth of today is to keep the dream alive. When your 6' x 8' cubicle feels like your 6' x 8' prison cell, keep the dream alive. When your recent pay cut contributes to your CEO's recent pay raise, keep the dream alive. And when you feel like giving up on the limitless possibilities that you see today, keep the dream alive. Do what must be done to pay the rent, but by all means continue to dream.

Although I haven't achieved my dreams, I remain an eternal dreamer. It's the one thing that keeps me going. Imagine a life without dreams or a life without a way to share the dreams that we do have.

"What's your dream?" Tapping my feet along the foot board of Cade's bunk bed, I question.

"Daddy," Cade pauses and shouts back to me. "Shrek!"

"That's right buddy." In my best Donkey voice, I reply "Shrek and Donkey on another whirlwind adventure."

"Daddy," Cade asks. "Who's Shrek like?"

"Shrek's like you buddy."

"Daddy." again he asks. "Who's Donkey like?"

"Donkey's like me."

"Yeah. Donkey's like Daddy."

With my head nestled upon Cade's Superman pillow, my feet continue to tap. "What's your dream buddy?"

An epic battle of action figures endures as I lie in bed waiting his reply. Still sitting on the floor, Cade inches back exposing ample amounts of butt crack. I watch as he lifts the joker from the crowd.

"Do you know how I got these scars?" He sinisterly questions.

"No," he replies in a bad ass Batman voice. "But I know how you got these."

Within moments, the wrath of Batman sends the Joker flying across the room adding to the many holes already plaguing our sheetrock walls.

"Cade," I attempt once more. "What's your dream? What do you want to be when you grow up?"

"What do you want to be?" Speaking of himself in the third person, Cade jumps to his feet in excitement. "You want to be Batman!"

"Well, that's a rather lofty goal," I tell him. "But let's see what we can do. Hey, maybe I can be Alfred. That way I can provide the tools that you need to be Batman."

"Yeah!" He stands proudly with his hands on his hips. "Cade will be Batman for Halloween and Daddy will be Alfred." Content with his Halloween costume choice, he rejoins the madness on the walnut floor. "Riddle me this...riddle me that"

"Cade..." determined to get an answer, I repeat my question. "What do you want to be when you grow up?"

"Daddy..."

"Yes buddy?"

"Who's Dora like from *Dora the Explorer*?"

"Ms. Leidy," I reply.

"Daddy..."

"Yes buddy?"

"Who's Diego like from *Go, Diego, Go!*?"

Knowing the answer Cade seeks I respond, "Mr. Carlos."

There's a brief moment of silence while Cade digs the Joker's head out of the drywall.

"Daddy…"

"Yes buddy?"

"Who would make a good Wonder Woman for Halloween?"

"Nelly Furtado of course."

My heart yearns for the day that Cade can share his dreams with me. Many nights I gaze from my bedroom window hoping to spot a shooting star. Lying still I pray. I wonder if the man upstairs can hear me. I wonder if He will ever grant me the peace of knowing that Cade will be all right; that my buddy will always have someone to look out for him. Slowly my eyes close and I wish.

Over the next few months I obtain a personal trainer certification. From noon until 1:00 pm I run a boot camp fitness class while Cade is in school. Fitness training is like recess from my daily household chores. Routinely, I encourage Julee to start a new hobby. Her last diversion outside of our home was belly dancing and that was over three years ago. I really do miss her belly dancing days. The tantric music and insane hip gyrations brought a new cultural experience into our home.

External hobbies are of no concern to Julee. Whereas, literature has proven to be all the escape that she needs. Hour after hour, her leisure time is spent reading. Made up faces in made up places, there really is no better getaway. Julee treats her books the same way that she treats a night on the town with cocktails.

"A glass of wine followed by a glass of water," she says. "The hydration prevents a nasty hangover and the pacing prevents a drunken spectacle."

When it comes to books, it's fantasy followed by fact. Reading fiction, she says, sparks her imagination. Non-fiction, on the other hand, provides valuable insight. Julee's friends often describe her as a free spirited woman walking through life just swinging her red purse. These would be the carefree moments when her head's in the clouds thinking of her favorite books. Little do they realize the weight of worries that she carries alongside that crimson handbag. Literature helps to lighten her heavy load.

Day in and day out. The same struggles. The same heartache. The same worries as the day before. A trip to the nearby Books-A-Million is Julee's definition of happy hour. A daring wizard, a brave young woman fighting oppression and injustice, a scientist on the verge of a medical breakthrough; these are the things that keep her red purse swinging high.

While Julee was pregnant it was light-hearted tales only.

"I don't want the baby to worry," she'd say.

From light-hearted tales to self-help with autism, Cade has had a big influence on the books that Julee reads. She often shares her books with Pat and Aunt Delores. Likewise, their love of books is shared in return.

"You'll just love this one," declares Aunt Delores. "It's very suspenseful and there's a lot of sex."

"Sounds great." Although uncomfortable talking about sex with her eighty-seven year old great aunt, she goes along.

"There's even parts about the oral sex," she continues. "If your uncle would have told me to put that darn thing in my mouth, I would have told him to go to hell."

"Aunt Delores!" Like a child, Julee covers her ears.

"Oh, you don't do the oral sex, do you?"

"Can we talk about something else?"

"Julee," Aunt Delores declares. "The penis is a very dirty thing, I tell you. I've washed many penises in my days of nursing and I've seen them all; the white ones, the black ones, the Spanish ones, and even the Asian ones. And they're all dirty; every last one of them."

In disbelief, Julee listens to her aunt's lecture on the male genitalia.

"And believe me, it's true what they say about the black ones. I tell you, there is no bigger penis than a black penis." Aunt Delores further elaborates as her hand gestures illustrate the length of the great black cock. "And how has Kelly's friend Pookie been? Oh, I just love him."

Eager to change the subject, Julee finds herself puzzled that penises somehow led to Pookie. "Pookie is fine. He'll be joining us for Thanksgiving dinner again this year with his kids."

"Oh wonderful. Tell him that I can't wait to see him."

Pookie has been spending every Thanksgiving with us in the Carolinas ever since Hurricane Katrina. Following the storm, he relocated to Austin, Texas. Unfortunately, his ex-wife and the children they had together were displaced in Atlanta, Georgia. One of the most devastating effects of Hurricane Katrina was the distance that it placed between loved ones. There were now over nine hundred miles between Pookie and his kids. On the other hand, the new job Pookie landed in Austin gave him the income that he needed to better provide for his family. Pookie had been a corrections officer in St. Bernard Parish, Louisiana for many years. He used to always tell me that working at the prison was like going to a high school reunion. Many long nights were spent reminiscing with the inmates / classmates. Unfortunately, the pay wasn't so good. It turned out that the same job in Travis County, Texas paid almost twice the salary.

"My plane just landed." He calls to tell me.

Upon receiving his call, I head out to the airport. It's a quick ten minute drive. Or in Prius talk: it's about forty-eight cents.

"OK. There you are." I tell him. "I can see you."

"Where are you? Are you sure that you can see me? You know that we all look alike, don't you? I'm standing next to the parking shuttle." Leaning over the curb, Pookie scans the rows of approaching cars.

"Yes, I see you. I am practically in front of you." Tapping my headlight switch, I signal to him.

"A Prius?" Surprised by my latest vehicle, he ducks his head and sits beside me. With his knees pressed against the dashboard he asks, "What happened to your last car? I liked that FJ Cruiser."

"Just trying to save some money," I explain. "This is the Prius C. It's the smaller version."

His hair brushes against the interior ceiling as he turns his head towards me. "I can see that."

"You know you can push the seat back." I inform him. As he reaches behind the seat to re-arrange his luggage, I explain to him my car buying experience. "It all started with that Nissan Armada."

"That was a nice car." He pushes back on his seat and stretches his legs the best that he can. At 6'4", Pookie's a rather tall gentleman. "There was plenty of room in that Armada."

"Sure it was nice." I agree. "And it was a great vehicle when company was visiting. But it was usually just me driving around and burning up gas at 11 miles per gallon. With the amount of driving I did between work, running errands and going back and forth to New Orleans, the gas was killing me."

Gas was priced at around $4.00 per gallon when I owned the Armada. My average monthly fuel bill was over $700.00. Determined to trade-in the Armada for a hybrid I went to the local CarMax. While there, a yellow Toyota FJ Cruiser caught my eye. It had a cool retro appeal and a manual transmission. My first car was a stick shift and ever since then I've had a fondness for manual transmissions. While the fuel efficiency of the FJ Cruiser was only 16 mpg, I justified the purchase by telling myself that I was improving my mileage by 5 additional miles per gallon – an approximate 45% improvement over the Nissan Armada. Needless to say, I drove off the lot in a yellow FJ Cruiser that day.

I really enjoyed that vehicle. I could throw my mountain bike in the back and just wipe down the interior when finished. Unfortunately, at 16 mpg I was still spending over $500.00 per month on gas. While working at the bank, the company offered a $3,000.00 incentive to employees who bought certain alternative fuel vehicles. That's when I decided to once again go car shopping. The Toyota Prius C was one of the most economical choices. My only reason for making the purchase was to save money, so it made the most sense. However, after test driving I just couldn't do it. I just couldn't see myself driving a tiny Prius C. Not wanting to give up my FJ Cruiser, I hopped in and drove home. Along the way, I stopped at the closest Starbucks. With a Caffe Americano and my cell phone's calculator, I did the math. Not only did the Prius have superior fuel efficiency, but it also operated on regular unleaded instead of premium. My gas bill would drop below $140.00 per month.

Continuing my conversation with Pookie, "I parked that FJ Cruiser, cleared out my stuff and went right back into the dealership. I asked the salesman to get me the Prius that I test drove. He asked if I would like to look at any other colors or options…"

"And I guess you didn't." Pookie interrupts.

"Nope. I just said, "Man it's a Prius. Just give me what you've got.""

I've been cruising around in my white Prius C ever since.

"And how's Julee and Cade?" Reclining back Pookie inquires.

"Doing well. Cade has come a long way since the hospital. Staying home with him has made a big difference." I continue. "What about Tyler and Summer? How are they doing?"

"Good. Tyler has gotten really good at football." Pookie's eyes light up as he talks about his kids. "But he's getting so big. That boy's almost 6' tall and he eats everything in sight… Summer, now she's still a tiny little thing… And she's getting so pretty. I don't think I'm ready for that."

"That's all right." I tell him. "You have a concealed weapon permit. When are we picking up the kids?"

It's a mid-afternoon, the Saturday before Thanksgiving as Pookie and I drive home from the airport.

"Tuesday," he replies. "We can take them back Sunday if that's all right."

"Absolutely. It's about a 3 ½ hour drive to Atlanta; or $15 in Prius talk."

"Damn! Maybe I need one of these."

We spend the remainder of our ride home in laughter paying homage to the first vehicles that we owned. Mine was a 1979 Datsun 210 station wagon. It had fake wood grain panels along the outside and Jheri curl stains on the vinyl seats and ceiling on the inside. The rusted wagon backfired every time I shifted gears and the worn out shocks made for a bumpy ride. Because of the occasional flames that shot out of the back, my father-in-law nicknamed my car the Batmobile. Although I never arrived in style with the Batmobile, I arrived nonetheless. I had friends with privileged lives that drove shiny new cars all thanks to their parents. However, many of my other friends had cars far more flawed than mine. I recall many evenings push starting Pookie's Pinto. The car killed every time that it idled and had a faulty starter to boot. I remember pushing his car through the drive through window of the neighborhood Popeye's. With biscuits and a box of chicken we ran behind the car. Once there was enough momentum, Pookie started the car by popping the clutch. With a little extra effort, his Pinto got us where we needed to go.

Forty-eight cents later, we arrive at my house. "Uncle Pookie!" Cade runs out to greet our guest.

"Hey Cade. Wow!" He exclaims. "You're even bigger than Tyler." It's amazing the changes that our bodies go through in our teenage years.

"Pookie!" Julee comes in for a hug. "I miss you so much."

"I miss you too Julee. More than you know. How's Michael and Pat?"

"They're doing well. They're looking forward to seeing you."

"I can't wait to see them. And how's Aunt Delores?"

Julee's eyes roll as she replies, "She's good. Funny, she was just asking about you."

"Really? I love Aunt Delores."

We have a great few days, Pookie and I. By Tuesday, Pookie is worn out. We've gone hiking every day so far. Crowder's Mountain is about fifteen miles from the house. Pookie's determined to work off the Tex-Mex meals he'd become accustomed to in Austin.

"We eat burritos all day long in Texas." He continues, "Breakfast, lunch and dinner! Sometime they give it a different name like quesadilla, taco or chalupa. It's the same shit, just a different tortilla. We even eat burritos for dessert."

Each day by the time that we reach the peak of the mountain, our shirts are off and tucked into our back pockets. The air always seems more brisk before the hike starts. Sweating profusely, Pookie looks over.

"You ain't tired yet?"

We climb a few extra steps to the summit, and there we stand looking in all directions. The view is always worth the effort. The rocky terrain at the top makes me feel like a kid in a playground. To our right is the Charlotte cityscape with its tall buildings stretching towards the sky. The steady take-off and landing of planes is evidence of a rapidly growing airport. To our left are the Blue Ridge Mountains. Although eighty to ninety miles from where we stand, they appear just a stone's throw away.

The trek downhill is so much easier. I spot a tall skinny tree and just can't help myself. Like a kid from the bayou, I climb until the narrow bark sways. With my hands and feet tightly grasped I breathe in the fresh fall air.

Fifteen minutes later, Pookie calls from below. "You gonna get your monkey ass down today? I'm getting hungry."

"All right.....All right...What are you in the mood for?"

"Anything other than a burrito is good with me."

Thursday soon comes and still no burritos. I also promised Pookie that there would be no turkey tortillas for Thanksgiving. The smell of fresh baked cinnamon rolls fills our house. Cinnamon rolls and the Macy's Thanksgiving Day parade have long been traditions of Julee's growing up. She's kept it going another generation.

The kids are soon awake and playing in the back yard. We watch through the window as they bury each other in the fallen leaves. The same leaves that I view as a chore, they view as a treasure. We have so much to learn from children.

Julee doesn't finish cooking until 1:30 in the afternoon. With just thirty minutes remaining until dinner, I clean the kitchen and set the table.

"I look a mess," she mutters and scrambles to the bathroom to get dressed.

Our Thanksgiving feast starts with Julee's Mardi Gras salad -- a Crescent City inspired dish named for its festive colors. The meal proceeds from there. By the time we get through the green bean and artichoke casserole, the shrimp stuffed mirliton -- a Louisiana bayou delicacy, the baked macaroni and cheese, sweet potato casserole, turkey with oyster dressing and gravy and freshly baked French bread; there's no room left for dessert. No big deal, there's still fifteen minutes remaining for the pineapple upside down cake to come out of the oven. Loaded with butter and brown sugar, it's one of my sister's most cherished recipes. Unlike my grandmother, Iris doesn't leave out any ingredients when sharing her recipes. Drunk on fat and carbohydrates, we lean back in our chairs.

"How's the medical practice going Michael?" Pookie queries.

"It hasn't been the same since we sold to the big corporation. I started the practice out of a desire to help people. Once we were part of the corporation it became too political, and so I left."

"I didn't know that. Did you retire?"

"No. I'm not ready to retire just yet. I decided to go to work for hospice instead."

"It seems like that would get depressing."

"It can be. But then again, it can be beautiful. Palliative care focuses on treating the person rather than treating the disease. Doing so, improves the quality of life for the patient and their families as well."

"I never really thought about that."

"This is what I mean when I say that it can be beautiful. I had a patient this past summer that was facing her final days. Her family wanted to give her one last Christmas. The room was fully decorated, Christmas tree and all. They even stood outside the window singing her favorite carols. Wearing heavy coats and wool scarves, they sang at the top of their lungs. It made me forget that it was mid-August and the temperature that day was over 100 degrees."

"Wow! That really is beautiful."

"It's so nice to see you Pookie." Aunt Delores chimes in. "I was just talking about you with Julee."

"She told me."

"You know, Julee's mom, Janice used to be crazy about you."

"I really miss Ms. Janice." Pookie says with a frown.

Julee's mom passed away of a massive heart attack three years before Cade was born. She was an amazingly loving woman and Aunt Delores was right. She truly did love Pookie.

Glancing over the table and thinking of loved one's past, I'm reminded of how much I miss the kid's table. The kid's table was filled with laughter. Never was anything serious discussed. You could belch and fart all you wanted. And there was always cookies and cheap frozen pumpkin pie. Excusing myself, I joined Cade, Tyler and Summer and the four of us had a blast.

It's amazing what a smile can do for the digestive system. Before long we're all craving Iris' cake and a cup of coffee. While passing around the dessert plates Aunt Delores leans over towards me.

"I sure do love that Pookie." Adoringly she gazes at him. "You know, he doesn't act B-L-A-C-K."

Later that night, while eating the remaining frozen pumpkin pie and playing in the leaves, I apologize for Aunt Delores's comment.

"Are you kidding?" Throwing a bucket of leaves over my head, Pookie replies. "That doesn't bother me at all. I love that woman. I love that she says whatever is on her mind. She always makes me feel like family."

"Well you are definitely family."

"Besides," he continues. "We all know that niggers can't spell."

On that note, I lean back and bury myself as deeply as I can into the dried foliage. Blowing swiftly I clear the area above my face. Surprisingly, it's quite peaceful. Lying still, I enjoy the beauty of the twilit sky. With me buried in leaves and Pookie finishing the last of the pumpkin pie; it truly is the best Thanksgivings ever.

Chapter 8

Homesick

Lying on my side, I tuck my hand under my pillow. All is silent.

"No chainsaws." I think as I roll to the right.

Missing are the sounds of karaoke and banging cabinets. With no coffee brewing, I know that Brett is fast asleep. For it's not yet 5:00 a.m. In a fog, I find myself drifting towards the kitchen.

Only it's not our kitchen. The Colonial wallpaper and avocado green appliances bring me back to my childhood home.

"Did I wake you?" Closing the louver doors to the laundry room, Mom turns around.

"No…I mean yes." Not even sure that I'm awake I stutter, "N…Nn…No."

"Would you like some coffee?"

"No thanks." Shaking my head, I smile. "Brett will be making some soon." Watching the care that she takes with our laundry, I let her know how much I miss her.

"I miss you too Sweetie. I know that you have a lot of responsibility now." A tear falls on my *Six Million Dollar Man* t-shirt as she gently folds the sleeves. "You may be many miles away, but you'll always be close in my heart."

Clearing the lump in my throat, "Maybe I'll have that coffee now."

I remember Mom's first Mr. Coffee machine. Using technology, the new coffee maker brewed a better tasting beverage. Unlike our old percolator, Mr. Coffee brewed at an even temperature preventing the coffee beans from burning.

By the time the last drop falls, we'd already shared a lifetime of memories. "I'll come visit soon." It was always calming to look into her eyes. "I promise."

Startled by crashing sounds and abrupt clatter, I find myself once again in my bed. Rolling back to the left I notice the time. It's 5:00 a.m. and Brett's scattering about the kitchen in his usual manner. Right away I know that it's not a dream.

"Hey, would you stop making all that noise?" Brett queries in his best Tramp voice. With the dog observing him, he continues, "People are trying to sleep."

Brett gently tugs at his Beavis and Butthead Christmas pajama pants as they fall below his rib cage. No one can pull off an electric guitar and holly wreath pattern quite like he can. With a matching Beavis Claus t-shirt he fixes the perfect cup for his outrageous sweet tooth -- a splash of peppermint mocha creamer and 5-6 teaspoons of sugar.

"Ahhh," Brett sips.

Marching to his room, his large rump shakes. The fleece bottoms gather tightly between his butt cheeks. Tramp follows behind lapping up the sugary splashes that Brett leaves trailing along the walnut floors.

There's a chill in the air as I debate getting up. On cold winter mornings I dread rolling out of bed. Conflicted with remaining under the blanket or getting up to raise the thermostat, I wave the TV remote. Larry Sprinkle on NBC is pointing to various parts of the state. No matter where he points, it's frigidly cold. Amused by a meteorologist named Sprinkle, I laugh silently to myself.

The rain and snow make for slick roadways. One of the best things about snow in the south is that the city shuts down. Don't ask the many northerners that live here about this. They bitch every time that it happens.

"You people from the south don't know how to drive in the snow." Distraughtly they moan. "That's why everything closes."

Despite their strategic snow driving abilities, I find the northerners' griping hilarious. Watching Mr. Sprinkle, I let out a huge cheer. School will be closed for a snow day. Eager for Cade to wake up, I run out the back door. Wearing nothing but boxer shorts, I shiver as I prep the downhill slope in our back yard. The sudden drop behind our shed is the perfect accompaniment for our red plastic sled.

"What are you, twelve years old?" Julee shouts through the glass door. "Get back in here and put on some clothes."

Determined to have some fun before it all melts away, I run inside to get Cade. To my surprise, he's not in his room. He's sitting quietly on the couch and gazing out the front picture window.

"Do you want to build a snowman?" Ready to play, I ask.

Sadly I watch as he misses out on the winter fun. "I am sure he would love to build a snowman," I think to myself. Unfortunately, the barometric pressure changes that accompany snow days are no fun for Cade. Cloudy, rainy and snowy days have become migraine triggers as well.

He continues his gaze as the children slide downhill. How I wish that he would go outside and play with me. I miss the days of Cade and me playing in the snow. We would run around the yard without a care in the world. You'd swear it was the Fourth of July. The Fourth of July with a snow ball fight; now what could possibly be better than that?

I hate watching him suffer. He's my best buddy. "Do you want to build a snowman?" Again I ask. His pale complexion and tired eyes tell me otherwise.

December is proving to be a rough month. It's been filled with rain and like the weather, Cade has spent most of his days gray and dreary. But then again, there were those few cherished days in between when the smile on Cade's face said it all. It was as though he became alive in the sunlight. The clear Carolina blue skies brought hope. Free from pain, he was eager to get out and appreciate life. As a parent, I long for those days.

I long for the days when he can live without chronic pain. It hurts thinking that on top of all of my son's many hurdles, he has to be in pain as well. There's a solution somewhere out there and one day we will find it. Until then we'll keep embracing the good days and powering through the bad. Although Cade has many challenges, I've learned to count my blessings. I know there are others that have it so much worse.

I also know that there are others that take far too much for granted. These are parents that I am talking about. Having a child requires sacrifice. Having a child with disabilities requires greater sacrifice. Things once important become insignificant. Money gets sacrificed. Social lives get sacrificed. Careers get sacrificed. I would sacrifice life itself for my son. Therefore, it pains me to hear a parent complain about sacrificing 'time' for their child.

So, here we sit, another year's almost over and a new one's just around the corner. With a new year comes new promise. I look forward to the progress that we can make in the coming year. Reflecting back over this past year there were many dark days indeed. It was in this darkness that we found strength.

Somehow we found strength. I just don't have the strength to watch my son looking gloomily out of the window any longer. Layered up, I head out into the winter wonderland. The glistening blanket of white gives way to my heavy footsteps. Like an explorer I search. Much of the snow has become icy from melting and refreezing. I continue searching. The ground cracks as I pace the yard. I stop for a moment to take in the beauty. Growing up in southern Louisiana there was always something magical about snow. "How magnificent," I think as I admire the natural splendor. My other thought -- "Damn! My feet are cold in these slippers." Slowly I turn to make my way back and there it is. A mound of the white stuff is left piled in the shadows of the shrubbery. And it's still soft and fluffy. With my bucket full I march back into the house.

The crackling of the fireplace is relaxing. With my warm smile and cold feet I sit next to Cade on the couch.

"Hey buddy," I hand him my bucket of snow. "Do you want to build a snowman?"

The two of us sit around the kitchen table, my buddy and I. A couple buckets later and our creation comes to life. At just under twelve inches tall, we make one bad ass little snowman. Looking out the window I notice the branches of the Dogwood tree. Heavy from the snow and ice they swoop just above Julee's Birdgirl statue. Julee fell in love with Birdgirl while reading John Berendt's *Midnight in the Garden of Good and Evil*. To surprise her, I bought her a replica. Dragging the concrete sculpture across the yard was no easy task. It wasn't until several days later that she finally noticed. Swinging her red purse, she held her head high as she walked happily by. "Oh my God! It's Birdgirl." She turned around in awe.

I smile as I continue looking out the window. Thinking out loud, I tell myself, "I guess I have to get out there and cut that branch back."

"What do you need to cut?" Julee asks as she approaches from the kitchen.

"One of the branches on the Dogwood looks like it may snap."

"But I love that tree." She sighs.

"It's leaning right over your Birdgirl statue."

"Well you better get out there and cut that shit down then!"

By the time the weekend comes the branches are neatly cut back. Tracking mud from the wet ground I stomp my feet and leave my shoes at the back door. I grab a pair of fuzzy socks and glide my feet across the floor. The music coming from our bookshelf stereo is joyful and merry. Cade found the remaining Christmas decorations that we stored away and it looks like the North Pole has exploded in our living room.

He didn't stop until every last ornament was hung. Just like the Dogwood I just trimmed, the branches of the Christmas tree are heavily weighed down. With my Shop-Vac humming I clean away. There's not an inch of the room that's not covered with pine needles and glitter.

"Daddy," Cade calls out. "Ten days 'til Christmas."

I stand there silent for a bit, my thoughts are muffled by the roaring vacuum. Bending over I reach for the mound of pine needles surrounding the tree.

"Merry Christmas!" I shout as I throw the needles into the air.

Later that evening, as I sit in bed picking pine needles from my hair, I lean towards Julee. "Do you realize it's only ten days until Christmas?"

"Serious?" Wondering how the holiday creeped upon us, Julee continues. "We better get cracking on Cade's list."

"I will take care of it Monday. No need to fight the crowds over the weekend."

"I didn't even get you anything yet." Like a monkey searching for fleas, Julee picks the pine needles still tangled in my hair.

"Don't get me anything. We don't need to spend the extra money." Thinking of Cade's wish list I continue. "I mean, have you seen Cade's list lately?"

Cade creates his wish list from flyers received in the mail. There's none better than Toys "R" Us as far as he's concerned. With scissors in hand, he jaggedly clips. Then, with a touch of hope and a ton of glue, he transfers these images onto a sheet of cardboard. By the time Christmas arrives, it isn't uncommon that his collage has grown several inches tall.

"I know." Julee laughs. "It's piled so high that he actually has packaging tape holding it together. And you're right," she agrees. "We should probably just focus on Cade and Brett this year."

Brett's eternally twelve, so there's no skimping on his gifts neither. Needless to say, his list can get rather extensive as well. I pull a pad from the kitchen drawer where Brett keeps it stored.

- the latest *Rock Band* game for his Sony PlayStation
- fresh underwear and socks
- a new karaoke machine
- various heavy metal t-shirts and CD's

These are just a few of the items that he scribbled down. Nothing says "Merry Christmas" quite like the screaming demonic tones of a death metal smash. I close the drawer as Brett walks by.

"Hey you twing-ling-ling-ling-ling." Looking my way, he opens the refrigerator, "Where's the egg nog?"

"I didn't buy any."

"Really?" The look of disappointment is evident on his face. "It's OK... I'm not mad." Shaking his head he marches back to his room.

Laughing I ask him, "What's a twing-ling-ling-ling-ling anyway?"

"Oh," he pauses and continues. "It's a tote."

The following Monday morning I place a spaghetti squash into the oven. In anticipation of holiday overeating, it's low carb in between. Dusting the shelves, I pick up a sparkling pink frame. It's a picture of me, Cade, Pookie and his kids. The goofy photo makes me smile. While strolling the Riverwalk in San Antonio, Texas, we spotted a kiosk of sequined hats. With each of our heads adorning a different colored hat, we struck a pose that would make Derek Zoolander proud.

I continue dusting while sounds of New Orleans fill my headphones. Listening to Harry Connick Jr's version of "I'll be Home for Christmas" makes me homesick.

"I've got to visit Mom and Dad soon." I think to myself.

My recent dream was so very vivid. I remember the yellow and white gingham pattern of Mom's old coffee maker. I remember how it clashed with the Colonial wallpaper. I remember my father teaching me how to hang that wallpaper at an early age. And I remember everything clashing with the avocado green kitchen appliances. That was a time; however, when appliances actually lasted long enough to go out of style.

Finished with my dusting, I move on to the floors. Back and forth I work the mop. With a steady eye on the clock, the floors are cleaned. It's time to tackle the mall. Calling Julee along the way, I give my progress report.

"You know, you don't always have to do so much." Sighing, she lets me know.

"I just don't want to feel like a dead beat staying home."

"Nobody would ever accuse you of being a deadbeat." She assures.

Weekdays make me feel rather useless. Julee has work, Cade has school and I have the desire to prove that I'm not a slacker. The house, on the other hand, has never been cleaner. We're smack in the middle of holiday season and Christmas is undoubtedly Cade's favorite. He enjoys the many merriments of the holidays. From the vibrant colors and cheerful songs, to the festive lights and joy shared by all.

Christmas morning as Cade lies in bed, visions of sugar plums are far from his head. The last of his gifts are placed under the tree and out of the house I scatter. With moves I learned from a James Bond movie, I sneak past Cade's window. Trying my best to keep quiet, I grip my sleigh bells tightly.

Silently, I wait for the perfect moment.

"Ho! Ho! Ho!" I shout as my sleigh bells ring out loud.

Just like clockwork, Cade's feet are set into motion. There's a magic I can't describe in the way that he still believes. Watching him, I recall the joy that I once had in believing; long before logical thinking spoiled the magic.

I don't remember exactly how old I was, but I know that I was younger than Cade. It was Christmas Eve and my brother Darrin,

Mom and I sat in the car waiting. Christmas Eve at Aunt Gloria's house was by far my favorite family tradition.

"Is Dad taking a crap?" Anxious to leave, I loudly asked.

"Kelly Jude!" Disapproving of my language, Mom continued. "Watch your mouth. It's Christmas."

"Well what's taking him so long?" I questioned as I jumped out of the car. "I'll go get him!"

"Get back in this car!" My mom frantically yelled.

Opening the front door to our home, I froze in utter shock. There were two Huffy bicycles surrounding our Christmas tree that weren't there before.

"Santa must be getting a head start," I thought to myself.

In awe I observed the shiny new bikes. My hands gripped the chrome handle bars as I saddled the elongated glittered seat. With my foot resting atop the left pedal, the same pedal that would go on to beat my shin relentlessly, I imagined racing past my friends to victory. A cracking sound from the hallway garnered my attention and so I tiptoed towards the clatter.

"Wow!" Covering my mouth, I realized that my thoughts had escaped me.

Right there, right at the foot of our attic ladder, Santa left his sack behind. A lawn and leaf garbage bag; the same type we use when cutting the grass and it was filled with lots of wrapped presents. Debating if I should dig in, again I froze. The sound of footsteps above my head could only mean one thing.

I watched as the shadowy figure approached. Just like in the books that I've read, his belly jiggled when he laughed. Quickly I turned. Excited yet frightened, I wasn't sure what to do. Keeping one eye on the attic opening, I hid behind the doorframe. Shaking as I stood there, the pieces suddenly came together. While we were in the car waiting and my dad was in the bathroom, Santa must have slid through the attic vent. After all, like most of the homes in my neighborhood, there was no fireplace for him to make his traditional entrance.

"I'd better go." Again my thoughts escaped my mouth.

Quietly as possible I tiptoed back to the front door. Then, as I reached to turn the knob I heard an all too familiar sound. Either Santa Claus developed a smoker's cough or in the attic was jolly old Saint Dad.

Later that same evening, while nibbling on roast beef finger sandwiches and bite-sized muffalettas, my cousins gathered around me. I had a yearning to share my discovery and Aunt Gloria's Christmas party provided the perfect opportunity.

Boy do I miss her parties. Aunt Gloria had a knack for bringing the family together. She also had a knack for shrimp salad. Finely diced with just the right amount of crunch, no one could duplicate her shrimp salad. Aunt Gloria's party foods were among the most sought-after recipes along Bayou Rd.

"Keith," I called for my cousin's attention. At only three months apart in age, Keith was my closest cousin. "There's no such thing as..."

"Tutti Frutti," Dad approached singing his usual greeting to my cousin. Keith and I were always close. Although Keith dated girls and periodically spoke down on homosexuality, I always knew that he was gay. My father, on the other hand, was somehow shocked when Keith came out as an adult.

"Seriously Dad?" I questioned him. "You always called him Tutti Frutti."

"Yeah, but if I knew that he was really gay, I wouldn't have done that."

For the better part of the next hour, Dad and Keith kept the rest of us in stitches. There was an unlikely camaraderie between those two. Throughout our time spent in laughter, I waited for the right moment. We kids had been lied to for all of these years and the truth about Santa Claus must finally be told.

Christmas tree illuminations reflected from the sparkling terrazzo floors. Aunt Gloria's house was always spotless. Perhaps it was due to Maw-Maw Tonia's rigorous buffing. Ever since I can remember, Maw-Maw Tonia has been a part of my aunt's household. Cooking and cleaning gave her a sense of purpose. I never really understood that until I became a stay at home dad myself.

Through the flickering lights, Mom's shadow appeared along the floor. Tipsy from the adult punch bowl. Mom reached down for her purse. Tucked away was a poem that she wrote for my grandmother.

"What I like best about the holidays," kicking off her shoes she continued, "is spending time with…"

Giving way to the lustrous sheen, Mom's nylons slid across the floor. I hadn't heard a sound like that until years later in 1996, when the first *Tickle Me Elmo* was introduced. With her rosy cheeks, she laid sprawled out along the floor rejoicing in holiday cheer. My father quickly tended to her and so I seized the moment.

"There's no such thing as Santa Claus!' I shouted. "I don't know why they do it. I mean who do they think they're fooling? Last year I saw where they hid the gifts. Then, when I visited Santa I told him exactly what I wanted. Since my mom and dad were standing next to me, I had to mention the things that I saw in their closet. And do you know what I got? I got the same things that I saw in their closet."

"But isn't that what you asked for?"

"Yeah, but I only asked for them because I knew that's what I was getting." Determined to set the record straight, I told them what I saw in our attic earlier that evening.

"Really? You mean Uncle Casie is Santa Claus?"

The good news is I didn't ruin anyone else's magic. There were just as many believers when I left the party as there were when I arrived. Anxious to get home, it was a long and restless ten minute drive. For I have seen the end of the rainbow and I knew that there were two bicycles atop that pot of gold.

Returning back to our driveway, I once again jumped out of the car. Moonlight filtered through the tall Magnolia tree as I raced towards the door. The evening mist trickled down the leaves as I brushed past Mom's azalea bush.

"Did you see that?" Pointing to the sky, my father looked up in bewilderment.

"See what?" I stepped out to take a look.

"A streak of light just took off from right above the house."

To amuse my dad I went along. "Oooh, what if it's Santa Claus?" Condescendingly I queried. "What if he came while we were at Aunt Gloria's house?"

Opening the door, again I froze. Gone were the treasures that surrounded our tree, replaced by a lousy note. A note from the big guy himself...

> If you don't believe...
> then you don't receive.
> - *Santa Claus*

"I believe! I believe!" Dropping to the ground I pleaded.

Drifting back to Christmas present, I'm reminded that indeed it was a joy to believe. For the better part of the afternoon, Cade is playing with his new toys. In the dining room the rest of us remain bloated on bread pudding. My sister prepared Christmas dinner and like most southern women, Iris over did it. Both Iris and my brother-in-law SJ were spending the holidays with us. Knowing that Iris was cooking we did the only logical thing. We bought larger dinner plates.

"I think that was the best gumbo I've ever eaten." Aunt Delores gently pats Iris on the back. "How have you been Sugar?"

"Oh, I've been good."

The kitchen sink is piled high with our dirty new dishes. Iris squeezes the handle of the stainless steel spray hose. Although the manufacturer says that the dishwasher can handle it, Iris says otherwise. Lightly rinsing, she places the dishes to the side.

"Here," Aunt Delores continues. "You rinse and I'll load the dishwasher."

"Oh, you don't have to do that." Iris declares.

"Listen baby, we're going to get these dishes done together… You and me."

The two of them reminisce about life in St. Bernard Parish B.K. (Before Katrina).

"I tell you Aunt Delores, I haven't been the same since that damn storm." Rubbing her fingers along the plate, Iris recalls. "It was so nice having everyone close by. Kelly and Julee had just bought their new home a couple of blocks from me. I always pictured walking beside Cade as he rode his bicycle to my house." Wiping her eyes with her forearm, she continues. "'Go to Nana's house.' That's what he'd say. My brother Darrin would come over several times a week. And although my brother Larry never visited much, I was only a couple of miles away when he needed me."

"The thing that I miss most about the Parish," Aunt Delores sighs, "is that everybody knew each other."

Louisiana is divided into 64 different parishes. However, if anyone in southern Louisiana made reference to "the Parish" or as the natives called it, "da parish," they could only be talking about one place. St. Bernard Parish is part of the New Orleans Metropolitan area. Adjoining New Orleans on the western side and the bayou on the east, St. Bernard Parish has always been a unique community. Since its formation in 1807, the roads had only two directions. If you were headed towards the city, you were going "up the road." And if you were headed towards the bayou, you were going "down the road." The direction to take just depends on "where y'at."

Hurricane Katrina devastated St. Bernard Parish. The eye of the storm passed right through it destroying almost every structure in sight. Packing a surge of nearly thirty feet, Katrina lifted entire foundations sending brick houses crashing into neighboring homes. Located in the middle of the neighborhood, our house in the Lexington Place Subdivision of Meraux, Louisiana remained standing. However, the water line when the chaos finally settled was four feet onto the second floor.

Listening to Iris and Aunt Delores in the kitchen, I can relate to every last word.

"Cade would stay with me." Again, Iris wipes her tears. "We'd walk to the front of the neighborhood and get snowballs. I was there when that baby was born and now he's over 700 miles away."

"You just don't find people like the ones in the Parish. All my friends were there." Smirking at the size of our dinner plates, Aunt Delores pauses. "You know, I don't think I could ever go back and see it. I just want to remember St. Bernard the way that it was."

"They've been rebuilding the area but it's just not the same. Everyone is scattered now and that's just depressing."

"Come on, Sugar. Let's go outside and have a cigarette."

"But I don't smoke, Aunt Delores."

"Look, I'm almost ninety years old and sometime it's the only thing that calms my nerves."

Outside on our covered patio the two ladies sit, rocking in the chairs that I just picked up from the nearby Cracker Barrel. As they light up their cigarettes, they start a friendly debate -- a debate that only residents of St. Bernard Parish would truly understand. Two unfiltered Camels later they come to a mutual agreement. Rocky & Carlos had the best shrimp po-boys and Randazo's Bakery definitely had the best king cakes.

"It looks like Aunt Delores recruited a new smoking partner." I announce as I rejoin the others in the dining room.

"Good Lord," exclaims Pat. "My mom is such a bad influence."

"Apparently, she told Iris that it would calm her nerves." I say to Pat.

A sudden burst of laughter and Julee blushes.

"What's so funny cuz?" Pat queries.

"She told me how to calm my nerves and it didn't involve cigarettes."

"Oh! I am so embarrassed." Pat pours another glass of Sangria. "Should I dare ask what she said?"

"Well…" joining Pat, Julee fills her glass. "She told me about when her mom passed away."

Letting out a sigh of relief, Pat lowers her glass. "I was expecting something much worse."

"She told me that when her mom passed away she became really depressed. She said that she didn't want to get out and do anything. She just wanted to stay home to herself. That's when Uncle Herlon suggested that the two of them should have 'the sex.' She said at first she really didn't want to have 'the sex.' But, then later decided, 'You know what? I'm going to have 'the sex.' You and Kelly sure have a lot to deal with. You should both go have 'the sex' together. You'll feel better, Sugar. I promise.' She then finished by telling me how happy she was that she listened to Uncle Herlon that day."

It didn't take Pat long to finish an entire pitcher of Sangria following that story. Some stories just go better with booze. My family's Christmas may not be the type that you'd see in a Lifetime Channel movie, but I wouldn't change it for anything.

Chapter 9

Forgiveness

The dawn of the New Year has come and gone. We'd just finished the last of the holiday leftovers remaining in our freezer. My pants are feeling tight and I'm committed to extra cardio. It's shortly after midnight Friday. Exhausted from a rough evening with Cade, I take to social media.

> "So this is what autism looks like after midnight. Allergies are off the chain. Migraines combined with sensory overload. He's been chewing the shit out of his lip and his back is bleeding from scratching so much. Cade is pissed off and he wants me to know how fucked up this life is. Therefore, I'm running around the house to get away from him so that he can calm down. He won't hit anyone other than me. He's broken glass frames throughout the house. There's glass everywhere. There's blood splashed all over the furniture, ceiling and walls. He cut his hand and when he tries to hit me the blood goes wherever it may. Not to mention he shredded the shirt that I was wearing and I looked pretty damn good in that shirt. Although I feel myself losing faith when shit like this happens I refuse to give up. Nothing hurts more than knowing your child is hurting and there doesn't seem to be a fucking thing that you can do about it. Sorry about the profanity but fuck, fuck, fuckity, fuck. I've got him in the tub now and gave him a migraine pain pill. Soon he'll be rested and in a few hours we'll move on like nothing ever happened. I love you guys. Just know that if things are messed up and you feel like your life sucks, be assured

you are not alone. Let's make the best of this thing together. After all, misery loves company."

Having a child with disabilities, you quickly learn the power of forgiveness. Holding a grudge is a sign of weakness. If that's who you are then this life will destroy you. It takes strength to deal with this on a regular basis and it takes strength to forgive. We all have our burdens to bear, yet we all have the power to forgive. I love my son and holding back forgiveness means holding back love. Below is a post that I made the following afternoon.

"Julee took Cade to Urgent Care for his allergies today. He's now playing with his Batman and Superman toys and I'm loving it. Thanks to everyone for your outpouring of love and compassion. You guys rock!"

Sharing our experiences is important to me. I remember many late nights surfing the web looking for answers. I knew that there had to be others dealing with the same madness. It was the words of fellow autism warriors that provided the most hope. Google became more than just a search engine. It became a lifeline. And while many stories brought promise, there were those that brought despair.

Reading people's tragedies, I'm reminded of the phrase, "God never gives you more than you can handle." Honestly, I never really understood this phrase. After all, the very definition of suicide is people who were given more than they could handle. Life is hard. Even the most prized fighter meets an unbeatable adversary. It's understandable to just want to give up. However, when it comes to my son I will never give up. I will fight until the bitter end. And while some sayings I don't understand, here's one that I do.

"When life gives you lemons make lemonade."

I get it and here's my message to God: I thank you for giving me this life and I appreciate the strength that you've given me. But my boxing gloves are wearing down and I'm sick and tired of lemonade.

"Stay positive," I tell myself. "Search for the underlying beauty."

Living with autism is tough. However, the love that I have for my son is immeasurable. That boy amazes me every day. That "boy" is now bigger than me. And although he possesses the physical characteristics of a grown man, he remains a small child. His child-like nature prohibits him from seeing things in a vulgar or profane manner. And although his innocence is truly a thing of beauty, it makes teaching him a whole lot more challenging.

Here's an example for the ladies:

Imagine listening to your favorite tunes in the bathroom while applying your makeup. Your teenage son enters the bathroom. Now imagine him dropping down on the toilet and taking a big steaming dump. Then, as he's squeezing out a brown hand grenade, he starts asking you about Disney's *Aladdin*. Although innocent, it's completely inappropriate.

"Stay positive," I tell myself. "Search for the underlying beauty."

And here's an example for everyone else:

We're seated at a booth enjoying our burritos. It was a typical Monday evening and that means only one thing in our household – it's Moe's Monday. We've been going to Moe's every Monday for the past several years. Brett would have a tantrum if we missed Moe's Monday. There's nothing more pitiful than watching a forty-five year old man having a panic attack over a burrito. And offering Brett Moe's on a Tuesday is no consolation, so Moe's Monday it is.

We were finished eating and I sent Cade to the waste can to empty our plates.

"I'll get it." He shouted.

A plastic wrapper from one of the straws blew off of Cade's tray. As he bent over, roars of laughter and disbelief were heard. The entire rear section of the restaurant was given a view that they'll never forget. With the plastic wrapper in his hand Cade stood and pulled up his pants. He then took a few more steps closer to the waste can. This time the wrapper blew into the opposite direction.

"I'll get it." Again he shouted.

And just like that, the front section of the restaurant got to see exactly what they were missing. In other words, there was a full moon at Moe's last Monday night. Cade left the entire restaurant in awe. Yet, as far as he was concerned, nothing unusual happened. Although innocent, it's completely inappropriate.

"When life gives you lemons make lemonade."

Oh I get it. I really do. However, when life gives you a ten pound sack of lemons and only one teaspoon of sugar it's still bitter as hell. Feeling down, I recall the moments when Mom was at her breaking point. It was in those moments that she searched for the beauty in the world. Talking with her that evening, I'm encouraged to do the same.

"God's Great Creation"

I hear the music in the spring
The birds up in the air
They fill the world with sun shining
They haven't got a care
The little blue bird weaves his nest
He's snuggled in a tree
How lovely is the cardinal
His beauty I can see
The chirping of the mocking bird
He sings along with glee
The churning of the hummingbird
The robin is so free
The meadowlark is comfortable
The wren she plays a tune
How colorful the bobolink
The spring is coming soon
Come see the joy and beauty
God made them all for you
He's master of creation
He's also kind and true

Helen Melerine

Mom is right. There is beauty in the world. Sometime we just need reminding. The next morning I awake to a clear blue winter sky; the perfect day for a trip to the mountains with Cade. The Blue Ridge Parkway is only about an hour and a half away. And although fall is my favorite time to visit, the Appalachian Mountains are breathtaking year round.

"Come on." Curling my index finger I call Cade to the bunny slope.

"Hamburger Helper!" He yells.

A feeling of frustration is evident in his voice. Slowly Cade scoots his way across the snow.

With a smile on my face I extend my hand. "Let me help you."

Determined to do it on his own, he insists, "Cade do it."

And do it he does. He continues moving fractions of an inch.

"Mashed potatoes!"

Throwing my poles down, I laugh. I know that he's frustrated but Hamburger Helper? Mashed potatoes?

"Come on buddy. Let's go on the tubes."

There's a hill close by with inner tube slides. We kick off our skis and march through the snow. Despite the cold temperature it's a beautiful day. The birds flying high remind me of Mom's poem. And although technically the south, a ski resort isn't what I have in mind for a southern migration. As we make our way to the inner tubes, a group of eager teens scramble by. Their excitement is evident in the stories they share of surviving the Black Diamond. The elation in their voices makes me smile. With a feeling of guilt I think of how things could be if Cade were typical. Slowly my smile vanishes.

"Screw it," I think to myself. "We'll make our own Black Diamond."

Just like the lazy birds that refuse to go any further south, this will be our paradise. There will be some brave stunts performed on the inner tubes today! By far, Cade and I are faster than any of the preschoolers sliding on the hill. So what if it's not the Black Diamond. At least Cade isn't yelling random lunch items. And how would I feel not being able to verbalize my true feelings? Would I get pissed off and want to kick someone in the couscous? Or maybe tell them to go foie gras themselves?

We work up quite a hearty appetite on the slopes, my buddy and I.

"What would you like to eat, Cade?" I ask him.

"Food." He promptly replies.

"What kind of food?"

"What kind of food?" Repeating my question, he continues. "Let's see…um…how bout pizza?"

The drive home is filled with pepperoni, off-key car tunes and the following conversation on a loop.

"Dad, who's Dora like from *Dora the Explorer*?"

"Who, buddy?"

"Miss Leidy." Cade continues to his next question. "Dad, who's Diego like from *Go, Diego, Go*?"

"Carlos!" I answer.

"Yeah…Dad," he goes on. "Who would make a good Wonder Woman for Halloween?"

"Nelly Furtado."

I grin across to him. "You're my best friend."

Cade's musical mix keeps the party jumping. Justin Timberlake, Chris Daughtry, Timbaland and now the Bee Gees. The next small town is still several miles ahead.

"Bathroom, Dad."

"OK, we'll stop in just a few minutes."

"Dad." Squeezing his hoo-ha, again he lets me know. "Bathroom."

"Just a few more minutes."

"Bathroom!"

I know by the squirming in his seat that the bathroom can no longer wait. Pulling to the side of the forest lined highway, we make our stop.

"Bathroom, Daddy."

"This will be our bathroom." I explain. "We're going to pee like bears do…in the woods." Making our way through the trees I smile. "Just watch out for those damn tics."

Pulling down his trousers, he pees in circles onto the fallen snow. With his pants to his knees, I remind him, "Just the front, Cade. Just the front."

"Just the front." He repeats. "Nobody wants to see your butt."

"That's right buddy. Nobody wants to see your butt."

A sudden scream and Cade runs back to the car. Although cute and cuddly, squirrels scare the heck out of him. Pigeons too, for that matter. All I can say is, "Thank God that no cars are passing." How would I explain running behind a screaming teenage boy with his pants around his ankles and pee dripping down his legs?

We get home and Julee and I stand over the stovetop laughing. She continues stirring as I recap our day in the mountains. The kitchen smells of Creole seasoning as her wooden spoon blends the lump crabmeat and shrimp into an aroma that beckons me to dig in. And although I prefer crawfish in my etoufee, I never met a shrimp that I didn't like. One bite and I'm overcome with the spirit of the bayou.

"I GARONTEE!" Opening my mouth, my inner Justin Wilson escapes me.

The next morning, I look into the mirror and smile. It's important to celebrate the simple things in life; like not shaving when I don't feel like it. It's Monday and the only thing on my agenda is teaching my fitness class at noon. Because Cade stayed up late with his cousin, he's later than usual getting up for school. Fast forward to 11:00 a.m. and Cade's still lying in bed. At this point it's time to get moving.

Cade's not a morning person. Therefore, he needs to start the day at his own pace. In an effort to move him a little quicker, I strike a deal.

"Cade," I tell him. "If you hurry and get yourself dressed I'll take you to Toys "R" Us when you get back from school."

My intentions are good. I just hope I don't cause him unnecessary anxiety. With one eye on the clock, I watch Cade as he exits his bedroom.

"Wolverine, ahhhh!" Cade roars in his favorite Marvel hero t-shirt.

Joyfully, he marches towards the bathroom. Then, with a dollop of hair product (he prefers paste) he meticulously works his thick brown coiffure until it's just so. He grips his Iron Man toothbrush, and after a few brisk strokes his choppers are squeaky clean. It looks like clear sailing from here.

Unexpectedly, a loud outburst echoes from the bathroom.

"Cade, you need to be on time for school" he fusses at himself. "I am very disappointed in you."

There's no need to scold him. He does that on his own.

"No Cade, you're a good boy." I profess. "I'm very proud of you."

All is calm, at least for a moment. And then the scolding continues.

"Shame on you Cade." He rails in the third person. "You need to be on time for school."

Maintaining a tight grip on his toothbrush, he bangs it against the mirror. Then, with the fury of Iron Man's fist, the mirror is cracked and his toothbrush is snapped in two.

Increasingly angry with himself, his ranting intensifies. "You don't break things, Cade! How many times do I have to tell you?"

Clearly, it's time for superhero intervention. In my best Professor X voice, I coax the young Wolverine into pulling himself together. A few deep breaths later, he gathers his backpack and we exit the house. Strolling towards the car, we whistle a happy tune – the theme song to *X-Men: The Animated Series*. The look in Cade's eyes, however, tells me that he's still not pleased with himself. Throwing his back pack down, he stomps along our red brick sidewalk. With all the mighty force that his two hundred fifty pound body can produce, he continues pounding both feet.

"Would you like to stay home?" I ask.

"Go to school!" He screams and runs to the car.

The car door slams and he fires a spitting rampage from inside the vehicle. In an attempt to once again calm him down, I open the door.

"Would you like to go back inside for a little while?"

I let him know that we can go to school later. With the force of a championship linebacker, he pushes the door open so that he can slam it shut again. Standing along the line of scrimmage, my shin bears the brunt of the blow and I fall to the ground. Cade notices and what happens next is truly remarkable. The car door opens and with big tears, he looks me directly in the eyes.

"Look what I did." He cries. "I hurt you. I'm sorry Daddy."

Clearly and with great sympathy, Cade apologizes. Joining my shin, my heart immediately melts. Fortunately, I'm wearing jeans. I show Cade my leg and let him know that I'm going to be all right. Relieved but still mad at himself, the thunderstorm of spit endures within the car. I march back into the house, grab my raincoat and drive merrily to school. By the time we arrive, Cade is once again feeling content. The next time you're on the highway and notice a smiling driver wearing a raincoat in a car with a spit covered windshield remember this; there's always a reason to smile.

No doubt my leg hurts. It's quite bruised. However, hearing those clearly spoken words is worth every ounce of pain. With a slight limp, I make it through my fitness class. I get home, wait for Cade to arrive and just as promised, I take him to Toys "R" Us.

"Oooh." Pointing to the car next to us, Cade chuckles. "Hey old nun!"

He continues pointing and before long his chuckle transitions into roaring laughter.

"Hey old nun!" Again he shouts.

We sit at a traffic signal as the old nun slowly approaches from the right lane.

"Why hello there." Dressed in full habit, she rolls her window down. "What a lovely young man. What's your name?"

"Cade!" He shouts and continues laughing. "Hey old nun!"

I clutch my St. Jude medal and stare straight ahead.

"Hello Cade." Her rosy cheeks highlight her welcoming smile.

"Hey old nun!"

"Yes my child?"

Speaking of himself in the third person Cade advises, "You don't hit the old nun with a hammer."

Making the sign of the cross, I realize that he's referring to a scene from the Three Stooges reboot that he just watched.

"It's from a movie," I explain. "*The Three Stooges.*"

"It's not nice to hit the old nun." Cade laughs.

"No," she agrees. "That's not nice at all."

"Just how long is this damn light anyway?" I ask myself.

"Hey old nun!" Cade elatedly shrieks. "Old nun…"

The light turns green and I immediately roll up the window and accelerate. Cade rises upward with the movement of the glass extending his neck.

"Dad," he howls. "That old nun is funny."

We arrive at the toy store, father and son. We enter the building, Thing 1 and Thing 2.

"Cade." My voice echoes through a voice changing Darth Vader mask. "I am your father."

The clerk, a young man with acne prone complexion, appears to be a bit perturbed. Granted, his aisle is very neatly stocked. He continues straightening as Cade and I play. Extending my arm, I pass Cade a lightsaber. It's Luke Skywalker versus Darth Vader, good versus evil, store clerk versus man-child.

"Sir," his internal struggle breaks free. "Please don't do that."

My head quickly ducks dodging Luke Skywalker's vengeance. "Do what?" I ask.

"We have a rule against horseplay in the store."

"Just seeing if it works." I reply.

The clerk nods, meticulously straightens a few more items and then raises his eye brows. "Of course it works," he mumbles to himself.

Sadly, I observe him. What I see is a young man that's grown up too soon. A young man far too serious to be in a toy store.

"Do you own one of these?" I ask from behind my Darth Vader mask.

"No…" Pausing a moment, he glances my way. Briefly, I see something resembling a smile, but then he's back to tending to his shelf.

"It's a shame." I inform him. "You really should get one." Observing his work, I continue, "I can tell that you take pride in what you do… That's very admirable."

"Thank you." He replies showing it once more, that certain something that resembles a smile.

"I can also tell that the force is strong with you."

His smile breaks free in a tug of war with the bright green rubber bands fastened to the braces on his teeth.

"Honestly…" He announces. "I'm more of a Yoda guy."

Noticing Cade's spastic lightsaber twirling, he offers his assistance.

"May I?" He asks.

The Jedi master takes over. "This is how to properly hold a lightsaber in ready position." Repositioning Cade's hand, he continues, "Place your thumb right here on this slot. Now with a firm grip, make sure the lightsaber is pointing in an upward slant."

Awkwardly, Cade follows along.

"Now this is how to block your moves." He explains.

Demonstrating proper striking techniques, his weapon glides from left to right and high to low. And just like that, I'm sold on two new lightsabers. The best salesman, after all, are those that display passion in their product. A tour guide in love with his city, a car salesman with a flair for the road, a toy store clerk in touch with his inner child. These are the ones that close the deal.

"Finished your Jedi training, you have." The clerk announces in a fairly weak Yoda voice.

With a twist of his wrist, he disengages his lightsaber and gets promptly back to work. There's a newfound realization that his job can actually be fun. Nodding a sign of gratitude he moves on.

We exit the building; me, Cade, a couple lightsabers and a Darth Vader mask, and embark on our journey home.

"Dad…"

"What, buddy?" I ask as we board the car.

"Who's Dora like from *Dora the Explorer*?"

"Who, buddy?"

"Miss Leidy." He answers and then moves on to his next question. "Dad…"

"What, buddy?"

"Who's Diego like from *Go, Diego, Go*?"

"I don't know, Cade. Who's Diego like from *Go, Diego, Go*?"

"Carlos!" He replies with an obvious tone. "Dad…"

I turn my head and give him an inquisitive eye.

"Who would make a good Wonder Woman for Halloween?"

"Why Nelly Furtado of course."

"Yeah."

Chapter 10

Unconditional

"Oooh..." Walking towards the couch Cade murmurs. "You don't sit on the glass."

Like a bandit with a guilty conscience, Cade proceeds to give himself away.

"Now you broke it." He sighs.

Unfortunately, I know exactly what he means. Cade has been punching and breaking glass as a means of dealing with his headaches. Glass windows, glass frames, glass mirrors -- a happy home is a shattered home, I always say. Cade has a limited ability to verbalize and sometime it just feels good to break shit. I understand. However, just like that annoying algebra teacher we all hated, I'm determined to teach Cade a less destructive, less expensive and less dangerous way of coping.

- (A) Razor Sharp Edges + (B) Fists of Fury = (C) Catastrophe.

Concerned with the possibility of him severely hurting himself, last Thursday I Googled images of graphic hand injuries.

"This is what could happen if you continue to punch glass." Turning my head, I gagged from the grotesque images. "Do you want this to happen to you?"

The stunned look on his face told me that he finally got it. Or so I thought. After all, he did stop "punching" glass. Thursday we had two windows in need of replacement. This morning we have three.

"You don't sit on the glass." Again he sighs.

I follow my gut to the window beside Cade's bed and sadly my gut is right.

"I should have known he would try this." I tell myself repeatedly.

The logic being, if you can't punch glass just sit on it until it breaks. Here's how that unfolded.

Cade's allergies had been hard-hitting. Although springtime in the Carolina's is beautiful it can be quite brutal. "Brutiful" is a good word to describe it. It was a brutiful morning! Lying in bed I gazed at the blooming dogwoods. The dawn chorus signaled the start of a new day.

"You don't sit on glass." Cade warned himself between sneezes.

"Are you all right?" I opened the door to his room.

"Daddy," he continued. "You don't sit on the glass."

"No Cade. You don't sit on the glass."

The glossed look in his eyes signaled that a migraine was on the way. Determined to stop his headache in its tracks, I returned with two Excedrin and an allergy pill.

"Here buddy. This will help."

Confident that I prevented a major outburst, I Googled graphic butt injuries. Five more minutes of sneezing followed by five more minutes of stomping. Then all became calm inside Cade's room. Outburst avoided. Or so I thought.

Don't Squeeze the Spaceman's Taco

"Oooh... You don't sit on the glass. Now you broke it."

It's just a couple minutes past seven in the morning when Cade sits on the sunken cushion of our beat up couch. It too has become a punching bag of sorts. The remaining fragments of the insulated window illustrate a life of chronic pain. Slowly and carefully, I guide my index finger across the cracked surface. The tiny shards remind me of how fragile our lives can be. How quickly our comfort and well-being can turn into agony and our happiness into despair. My son has gifted me with unconditional love. If broken glass is my price to pay for unconditional love, then I'll bust out every damn window in the house and relish in the April breeze.

Parenting -- nobody said that it was going to be easy or inexpensive. The worry, the grief, the endless trips to Home Depot. Although my checkbook has been drained, my heart has been filled. My life before Cade was a flip phone. Convenient and tried-and-true, I had no need for anything else. No need whatsoever. After all, things were just fine the way that they were. I now have the ability to learn a foreign language, monitor my heart rate and find the nearest Starbucks right in the palm of my hand. Cade was the update that my internal operating system so desperately needed.

Unconditional love, what does it really mean? It means loving someone regardless of the physical and emotional scars that they have caused. It means loving them for who they truly are. It means loving someone even at their most unlovable moments. When you love someone unconditionally, you love them just because. Approaching Cade on the couch, I keep a stern face.

"Don't ever break glass again. Not with your hands. Not with your butt. Not with any single part of your body."

Silence descends over the room as I give him a menacing glare. Squinching his face as if he ate a Sour Patch Kid for the first time, Cade turns his head towards me.

"No..." He clears his throat.

Struggling to hold a mean mug, I'm laughing on the inside. That face that Cade makes does something to me. In my best drill sergeant voice, I demand clarification.

"Do you understand?"

"You don't break glass." Speaking of himself in the third person, he continues. "You might cut yourself. You might get blood all over the place. You might get your hand cut off... get your foot cut off... get your face cut off... get your ass cut off."

And for this lesson, I have Google to thank. What did parents do before the internet?

Mom believed in prayer. That if you prayed hard enough, He would hear you. And if not, it just wasn't God's will. For He had a plan. I on the other hand, believed that if He had a plan why ask for anything specific to happen. If it is indeed God's plan, why not just pray for acceptance of the outcome rather than the outcome itself. But I never questioned Mom. To her, prayer was sort of a magical thing. If you believed, then miracles abound. Perhaps that's not such a bad thing.

It's not a bad thing until you start sending money to the crooked preachers on TV. That's how Dad viewed it. It wasn't uncommon to find my mother kneeling before the television set on any given Sunday afternoon. With her palms pressed tightly against the wood grain console, she awaited the many blessings promised for her generous donations.

Dad wasn't big on church. He figured that as long as mom went, then she had the rest of the family covered. Nor was he big on small talk. Don't get me wrong. He truly loved the people in our neighborhood. He just didn't feel the need to chat on a regular basis. Vivian, on the other hand, was the most loquacious voice on the block. She lived in the house next door. While dad was a man of little words, Vivian was an entire encyclopedia of words. From A to Z, the simplest of conversations extended for hours.

"Yoo-hoo." Poking her head through the crack in our front door, Vivian let herself in.

In our neighborhood, one didn't wait to be invited in. One was always assumed welcome.

"I baked a batch of sugar cookies," she announced. "And little Chuck already ate over a dozen himself."

Barging into our kitchen, Vivian delivered her homemade goodness.

"Hey Vivian," Mom greeted. "Those look delicious. Why don't you join me for a cup of coffee?"

"Honey, I can use a cup of coffee. Do you believe that little shit ate over a dozen cookies by himself?" Vivian rambled as she laid her Chinet plate upon our countertop. "I said look here boy, let me take the rest of these cookies next door before your belly pops."

"Oh Vivian, that's very kind of you."

"It's nothing Helen. These are very simple." Reaching as Mom handed her a cup, Vivian continued. "You just mix some butter and sugar into a bowl."

Breaking from her recipe, Vivian took her first sip. "Needs a little more cream," she acknowledged.

"Then, you beat in your eggs and vanilla extract. Blend in the flour. Add a pinch of baking soda and baking powder." Taking another sip she sighed, "ahhh… just right."

Mom nodded as she mentally noted Vivian's recipe.

"You then make little balls with the dough, place them on a cookie sheet and bake them for about ten minutes at 375 degrees."

Vivian took another sip before noticing Mom's new draperies.

"I just love those curtains," she announced. "When did you get those?'"

"Iris bought those for me." Mom lovingly gazed towards her new curtains. "She got them from the JC Penney catalog."

"That Iris," declared Vivian. "She has such good taste. How is she?"

"She's doing well. I'm so glad that she moved closer. With her living just a couple streets away, I can walk right over when Casie gets on my nerves."

"Girl, I hear you. But doesn't she miss living up the road?"

"You know Vivian, Iris has her own car." A woman having her own car was something unheard of in my mother's time. "So she can run the streets whenever she feels like it."

"I'm surprised that you never did get your own car, Helen." Biting into the cookie that she just dunked, Vivian continued. "I don't know what I would do without my own car."

Vivian worked in the meat department at Schwegmann's supermarket. Her job gave her an independence that many of the women in our neighborhood envied.

Don't Squeeze the Spaceman's Taco

"I don't like to drive. It makes me so nervous. Or should I say Casie makes me nervous?" In my dad's grumpy voice, Mom moaned. "You're going to slow, Helen. The big pedal on the right, Helen."

Hysterically, the two ladies carried on impersonating my father.

"Baby, I needed that laugh." Vivian wiped the tears that ran down her cheek. "Have you been keeping up with the stories? I tell you, that's the worst part about this job. I just can't keep up with my stories anymore. I love the extra money, but I sure do miss *The Young and the Restless* and *The Guiding Light*."

Over the course of the next two hours, Mom and Vivian discussed soap operas, macramé plant hangers, the neighbor's new microwave oven, gallstones, oyster dressing, flower gardens, nail fungus and facial care. Vivian never did run out of things to talk about, she just ran out of time.

"Girl, let me get my ass back home so I can cook something for big Chuck."

There were two men in Vivian's life, big Chuck and little Chuck. Little Chuck was like a brother to me. Chucky, that's what I called him. Chucky and I did everything together. It's wonderful how friends can become family. And just as Chucky was my brother, Vivian was very much my mother. She was my fun mom. She was horror movies and popcorn, board games and Kool-Aid. Vivian was gin rummy and Swanson's TV dinners.

"Hey Casie." Vivian smiled as she exited our house. "We were just talking about you."

My dad had just returned home with some supplies for his boat. Tomorrow would be the first day of shrimp season in southeastern Louisiana. Shrimp season was an important time of the year as it provided Dad with the opportunity to put money in the bank and food on the table. Loyal and true, I accompanied my father on his boat. A day on a shrimp boat is a long backbreaking day. However, for some reason I enjoyed it. Hours before the sun came up we'd cast our first net. In anticipation of a big catch, I'd settle for a quiet nap. It would still be another hour or so before the real work began. A picking box of just about three feet wide extended across the stern of the boat. Curled up within this wooden box, my eyes closed and I drifted. The smell of the bayou encompassed me.

There was nothing Zen-like about that salt water soaked wooden box. However, I learned the importance of finding comfort amidst the discomfort. There's an unequivocal power that arises from our moments of stillness. Lying motionless and blocking out the world around me gave me the strength that I needed to for the workload ahead.

"We're gonna eat good today!" Dad yelled out.

With a firm grip on the nylon ropes, my torso pivoted from left to right. Rested from my picking box nap, I was a pint sized ball of energy. My muscles contracted as the net floated closer.

"Look Dad!" Excitedly, I pointed. "A dolphin."

"That's a porpoise." Dad explained. "Dolphins have a longer, pointy nose like you."

Crossing my eyes, I examined my nose. Left to right, I reached and pulled until the net was close at hand. Dad joined in and together we pushed the bountiful net far below the murky water. A powerful buoyant force thrusted the net back above the surface and together we emptied the catch.

Then, like déjà vu, we'd cast the net once more. Dad steered the small skiff through the familiar water channels and for the next hour or so, I sorted the harvest. Into the cooler, went the shrimp. Into the lake, went everything else. Steadily, I picked until the last shrimp was iced. Working quickly allowed me fifteen minutes of rest time. Leaning over the side of the boat, I filled my bucket with water. Five heavy gallons later, I swished away the remaining debris and back into the picking box I lay. Surrendering to silence, I curled myself up. Slowly, my eyes closed and I drifted.

Back to reality. It's a quarter past 5:00 a.m. and the continuous slamming of doors awakens me. Rolling out of bed, I follow my ears to the kitchen. Mr. Yang, the curious stray cat peers in through the glass panels framing our front door.

"What's with all the racket?" Yang appears to ask.

I turn towards the kitchen and notice Brett scrambling frantically about the room.

"Listen Kelly," in a state of frenzy he alerts me. "We're out of sugar."

"Sugar?" I ask myself as I stand before him speechless. "All this noise for sugar?" Shaking my head, I join Mr. Yang on the front steps.

"Well Yang, I guess we're out of sugar."

He stares at me a moment, this cat, then licks his paw and turns away.

"Listen Kelly," Brett opens the door. "I'm trying to fix my coffee and we don't have any sugar."

"You know Brett," sarcastically I reply. "I don't have any on me."

"Oh…" he continues. "That's OK. I'm not mad. And by the way, we don't have any flavored creamer either."

Yang too is shaking his head. Brett doesn't receive the acknowledgement that he seeks and so he closes the door.

"Sugar?" I sit quietly on the front steps.

Yang looks up at me, tilts his head sideways, then licks his other paw.

"I know…" Again Brett opens the front door. "I guess I'll have to go buy some… Maybe I'll go to Dunkin Donuts."

"That's a great idea, Brett." I concur.

Bored with our conversation, Yang strolls off down the sidewalk. Ten minutes later Brett exits the house. His jean shorts are pulled high parting his moose knuckle ever so slightly. I go back in and wait beside the picture window. Brett runs past along the driveway, I laugh and then glide across the floor to the kitchen. Staring at the shopping list on our refrigerator door, I grab a pen and complete the list.

- Sugar
- Flavored creamer

Struggling to keep my eyes open, my head slumps and I glide in my socks back to my bedroom.

A couple hours later, Cade and I leave for the grocery store. We return home to a tantalizing aroma that's billowing from the kitchen.

"Cade, do you smell those cookies?" I ask.

Together we march eagerly towards the stove. Everything remains just as it was before we left. Although the smell says cookies, the spotless kitchen says otherwise. A shimmering light from the dining room catches my eye.

"Homemade Sugar Cookies," reads the label on the jar.

"A candle?" I shake my head. "You've got to be kidding me."

Yang peers in through the dining room window and he too is shaking his head. Now craving cookies, we turn around and head back to the store.

Determined to make our home really smell like "Homemade Sugar Cookies" we return 30 minutes later with cookie dough and action figures. The oven is pre-lit to 375 degrees. In goes the baking sheet and the, "If you like homemade cookies, you'll love this instant shit" cookie dough. Cade plays with his new Hulk and Iron Man toys and I clean up the mess. As I turn the knob to the laundry room door, I'm aghast by the repugnant odor.

"What's that smell?" I ask myself.

The room reeks of cat urine. Yang and friends live outside, so I know that it can't be them. Determined to get to the bottom of it, I follow my nose. Cautiously, I lower my head as I sniff inside the trash can.

"Nope." I tell myself. "It's not coming from there."

"Maybe it's the recycle bin." I turn my head and sniff in the opposite direction.

Although a bit stronger, it's not quite the stench that I'm searching for. I march to the dining room table, grab Julee's candle, place it on top of the washing machine and close the door.

"Brett," I shout. "Would you please take out the trash?"

Brett has only a few chores to do at home. He feeds the dogs, gets Cade off the bus after school and takes out the trash.

"Yep," he replies.

While in the laundry room, Brett loads the washing machine, twist ties the trash bag and then exits the house. His skull and crossbones boxer shorts are pulled so high that they barely cover his butt cheeks.

Stomping his way to the shed he shouts, "I wish I was taking you to the trash can. You jawannadoob!"

"Yeah?" I take a jab back at him. "Maybe you should put yourself in the trash. You squinky squat!"

Smiling and mumbling, Brett makes his way to our outdoor trash cans. In the meantime, I lock the door and stand alongside with a sinister grin. As Brett attempts to turn the knob, he starts shaking his head.

"Ooooohhhh! You better open the door." He yells at me. "You tote!"

I stare at him for a moment through the glass pane. Revenge is a dish best served with milk and cookies.

"Oooooohhh! I'm glad that you're locked out." Tauntingly, I tell him. "You trot!"

We continue our exchange of made up words and then I let him in. He stomps his high top tennis shoes, bends over briefly and pulls up his mismatched tube socks.

"Now get out of my way." He smirks. "You dribble drot!"

He then marches to his bedroom, closes his door and brings Freddie Mercury back from the grave. *"Bohemian Rhapsody"* reverberates throughout the house in all of Brett's off key glory.

"Ding…" The oven chimes signaling that the cookies are done. Brett takes a break from his rock band arena tour and joins Cade at the table. While they enjoy their snack, I clean the remaining dirty dishes and toss my towel into the hamper.

Pleasantly surprised, I notice that the odor is gone from our laundry room.

"It must have been something in the trash can, I tell myself as I blow out the candle and close the door.

The next morning I gasp again upon opening the laundry room door.

"What's that smell?"

Determined to uncover the source, I start removing items from the laundry room one at a time. The first thing out is the trash can.

Sniff…sniff…sniff… "That's not it."

Next out is the recycle bin.

Sniff…sniff…sniff… "That's not it."

Dirty towels.

Sniff…sniff…sniff… "Not it."

Our laundry hamper.

Sniff…sniff…sniff… "Not it."

Brett's laundry hamper.

Sniff…sniff…

Quickly, I jerk my head back and I gag. What I thought to be cat urine is actually Brett's body odor. I dump his dirty clothes into the washing machine, add an extra scoop of laundry detergent and press the start button. I then light up the candle and close the door.

"Brett," I ask. "Are you out of deodorant?"

"Nope," he replies.

"Are you using it?"

"Yes," he pauses and slowly answers.

"How about soap or shower gel?"

"Huh?"

"Are you using soap when you shower?"

"Yes."

"Water?"

"Oh yes," he declares. "I always use water when I take a shower. Why?"

"Just asking. That's all."

I discuss Brett's hygiene with Julee. She's shocked to discover that the musky odor plaguing our laundry has been her brother.

"Oh no!" She exclaims. "People are probably calling my brother 'the stinky man'."

We stock Brett's bathroom with a new assortment of toiletries and it turns out to be a big hit. Brett really seems to enjoy his new products. The next time he walks by he's "Zestfully" clean. He retrieves his work clothes from the dryer and heads to his job cloaked in April freshness.

Later that night I receive a call from Brett. He just finished his work shift and his scooter doesn't start.

"I'll be there shortly to pick you up." I inform him.

Upon arrival we load his scooter onto my trailer and fasten the tie down straps. I start the engine, fasten my seatbelt and once again gag.

"What's that smell?" Rolling down my window, I turn to Brett and ask. "Did you use the new deodorant that we bought you?"

"Yes," he replies.

"Are you sure?"

"Yes," he pauses then answers.

"Well Brett, I hate to tell you but you've been really stinky lately."

"But I'm using deodorant..." He stomps his feet. "Really!"

The cool mist splashes over my face as we drive home. Although it's raining, our windows remain down. Once home, Brett starts his usual routine. He kicks off his work shoes, leaves them in the shed and puts on his favorite high top tennis shoes.

"It's back." I announce as I walk into the house.

"What's back?" Julee asks.

Brett comes in and goes straight to the shower. Meanwhile, Julee and I join forces to figure out the reeking mystery. With his new loofah and fragrant shower gel, Brett scrubs away.

"Could it be a change in body chemistry creating this awful odor?" Puzzled, we think of all the possible causes.

"I'm all clean." Brett announces as he exits the bathroom.

Squeamishly, I hesitate as I ponder my next move. Gazing over Brett's dirty clothes still piled on the bathroom floor, I know what must be done. Slowly, I lean forward and pick up Brett's shirt.

Sniff...sniff...sniff... 'That's not it."

Next up is Brett's pants.

Sniff…sniff…sniff… "That's not it."

Brett's underwear.

The very thought and I'm puking inside my mouth.

"It's just not worth it." I tell myself.

Holding my breath, I throw his briefs aside. The only remaining garments are his socks. I lift them, inhale and I'm nearly asphyxiated.

Dizzy and a bit light-headed, the pieces of the puzzle come together. Brett has been leaving his work shoes inside our shed. Mr. Yang and the stray cat crew have been entering the shed through the pet door on the side of the building. Brett's shoes are being used as a litter box and the socks that he wears are absorbing the cat urine. These same socks are the ones that have been contaminating our laundry room. The mystery is solved!

P.S.: I have a pair of black skid proof work shoes for sale…dirt cheap.

Chapter 11

Inclusion

What's the world like through the eyes of innocence? Somewhere over the spectrum I see the wonder. I see the wonder of a world not tainted by ignorance and hatred; where superheroes exist and fairy tales really can come true. Children give us a unique opportunity to regain this magic.

"Daddy," queries Cade. "What's Santa Claus going to bring you for Christmas?"

"Let's see," speaking of himself in the third person, Cade answers his question. "Santa will bring you Batman, Superman and Justice League toys."

"Wow Cade!" I exclaim. "You must have been a good boy. But it's not even summer yet."

"It's not even summer yet." Sadly he repeats.

Noticing Cade's frown, I affirm. "But Santa is always watching and you have been a very good boy."

"Yeah," he so proudly agrees. "Daddy, what does Santa bring you if you're nice?"

"What Cade?"

"A bag of toys." Joy beams from his eyes. "Daddy, what does Santa bring you if you're naughty?"

"What Cade?"

"A bag of poo."

Although physically an adult, Cade remains a child. Autism may have robbed him of an ordinary life but Cade has taught me extraordinary lessons. Throughout the past two decades Cade has been the most fascinating person I've known. He has been a superhero, explorer, spy and space ranger. His adventures were always alluring to a man that settled for a boring job in banking. I must admit, his space ranger days always kept me on edge.

Cade was just two years old and plotting travel to the far reaches of the galaxy. One small step for man became one giant leap from the couch. Moments later we found ourselves in the emergency room with a fractured arm. That night, while my astronaut was fast asleep, I did what most parents would do. I painted his cast to resemble the beloved Buzz Lightyear's arm. "Perhaps I should have gone with that annoying purple dinosaur," I thought as Cade shouted, "To infinity and beyond." Cade may have been sure of his ability to fly but I wasn't sure of my ability to explain another visit to the hospital. To protect him from the perils of space travel we turned the couch upside down.

With the end of the school year quickly approaching, I'm reminded of school years past. At the time, Cade was in the second grade at Arabi Elementary and we were noticing big improvements with his speech. Using visual cues, he was able to complete simple reading and math assignments. Individualized Education Programs (IEP's) are developed by school administrators and the child's parents. IEP's are required for all children receiving special education services. Meetings are held at least once per year to determine if the goals set for the child are being achieved. I will never forget sitting with Cade's teacher during that year's epic IEP.

"We've noticed something new with Cade," his teacher informed us.

"What is it?" Dreadfully, I asked.

"Well," she paused for a moment. "Cade has been saying a few new phrases."

Sounded great to me so far. "What's wrong with that?" I thought to myself.

"Well...," she continued. "He's been saying 'Oh damn!' 'Oh shit!' and my favorite 'Oh fuck!'"

Hard as I tried, I couldn't stop smiling. "What made him say this?" I asked.

"The first time that I noticed was after he dropped his pencil. Now every time he drops or bumps into something he lets it out."

"Wow!" I exclaimed. "So he's using it appropriately."

"Well it's never appropriate for a seven-year-old, Mr. Melerine."

"Ok," I chuckled while maintaining a serious face. "We'll work on that."

Cade's teacher and her aids were all wonderful. However, there were no autism designed programs within the St. Bernard Parish school system at the time. The only school I knew of that offered such a program was located in uptown New Orleans. The cost for tuition was well over $20,000 per year. There was no financial aid, no transportation and no after school care. One of us would have to quit working just to get him there and that was financially impossible.

Then, later that same year the unimaginable happened. Hurricane Katrina ravaged through southern Louisiana leaving miles of mass destruction. The winds of change carried us hundreds of miles away to North Carolina. Thanks to Mother Nature, Cade was now in a public school system that offered autism specific programs. Throughout his remaining elementary years, Cade attended school with typical children. Most of his day was spent in classrooms devoted to students with autism. His remaining time was spent in moments of inclusion. Inclusive classrooms place children with disabilities side-by-side with their non-disabled peers. Through inclusion children learn acceptance. Children are given the opportunity to realize that despite obvious differences, we're all the same. Instead of forming judgement and fear, the children develop friendships.

Years passed and the end of fifth grade was approaching. It was time to find a new school. Cautiously, we reviewed the middle and high school options available. Cade's teacher and several others highly recommended Webb Street School. Webb Street provided a learning environment for students between the ages of 5 and 22 with intellectual disabilities.

"At this age kids can become cruel," we were advised. "Mr. Melerine, if you send Cade to one of these other schools he will become a drug mule. However, at Webb Street he will be with his peers. He will be with those that understand and appreciate him. At Webb Street he can be himself."

Determined that Cade should never compromise being himself nor carry narcotics up his rectum, we enrolled him at Webb Street School. It was a happy place filled with exceptional children. The school protected the students from the perils of the outside world. At Webb Street being different was not only accepted, it was encouraged.

"Why would anyone want to harm such beautiful beings?" I often wondered.

The answer is "ignorance." Ignorance causes individuals to somehow feel that they're better than others. Ignorance doesn't see beauty in things that are different. Ignorance sees fear and fear breeds evil. What does evil look like? It's not zombie-like creatures with decaying corpses like you may imagine. That would be too easy. The vile stench would give it away. Evil lies in faces like yours and mine. Evil is all around us. We let it 'in' when we fail to see the beauty in God's creations. We let it 'win' through racism, sexism, homophobia and heartlessness.

Proudly, I stood guard with the army at Webb Street School. Together we fought to protect those persecuted for being different. If anyone thought that they were better than others for some pathetic reason, I had this bit of advice to offer, "You are not smarter than a fifth grader. One thing I've learned from raising a former space ranger is that on Playground Earth we're all created equal."

Equality – It should never be a goal to endeavor. Yet, just like the targets on Cade's IEP, it's something that we strived to achieve each year. Equality is a simple fundamental of being human. Ironically, it's something that we don't truly appreciate until we're faced inequality. It took me becoming the parent of a child with disabilities to fully understand this. And in a world of sickening inequality, I have become Cade's voice. Although I willfully embrace the responsibility, I certainly never expected it. You see, Cade started speaking at an early age. But sadly enough, that all changed one day.

When Cade was just nine months old my sister, Iris taught him his first word. "Nana." That's what Cade calls her. Then, with some effort on our part, Cade soon followed with "mama" and "dada." Things were going great for our new family. We had a beautiful new starter home; an amazingly well behaved baby and I had just started a new job where I didn't have to work sixty plus hours per week. I remember a conversation that I had with one of my co-workers back then.

"I was getting worried about my daughter," she informed me. "But her pediatrician assured us that she is progressing at a normal rate. The doctor said not to compare her to kids like Cade. Cade is progressing at an advanced level."

He really was. Cade was quite the chatterbox by his second birthday. "I love Nana most," "Give me cookies," "Let's watch Teletubbies." All this changed just six months later. Cade developed a high spiking fever out of nowhere. He began trembling and stiffened with sudden jerks. The convulsions continued and they looked like spasms or seizures. Immediately, we rushed him to Children's Hospital. Panicked, I dialed 911 along the way.

"My son is burning up and having convulsions!"

"Ma'am," the dispatcher tried her best to relax me. "I need you to remain calm."

Calm was not an option. I stormed through those emergency room doors cackling in hysteria. Only once Cade was admitted did I sit back and regain my manly voice.

"Your son is going to be fine," the doctor assured me. "Febrile seizures can be frightening but within an hour or so everything is back to normal."

Relieved, we left the hospital with our son and a bottle of Motrin. But things weren't going to be fine and slowly Cade vanished in silence. My world was suddenly cast into darkness. Everything went dark. My son was gone. Our happy baby boy was no longer using the skills that labeled him advanced. He wasn't even crying anymore. Crying is a baby's first form of communication. Any attentive parent can identify their child's many cries. I knew when Cade was hungry, sleepy or hurting. I knew when he wanted to be held. I even knew when he dirtied his diaper just by the sound of his cry. But Cade was no longer crying those familiar sounds. Cade's only sound was a piercing scream. And with every howl I scrambled to comfort him.

That's when we began hearing the word "autism" and I began thinking of all the reasons that it couldn't be autism. After all, individuals with autism are born that way. Not Cade, he was advanced. Individuals with autism avoid eye contact. Cade looked me directly in the eye with no problem. Individuals with autism tend to line toy cars in a single row and spin their wheels. Cade played with toy cars just like any other typical child. Just to prove it, I bought more and more toy cars. I raced those toy cars around the room until my knees scabbed over. But no matter how much I denied it, Cade had autism. What could have brought on the sudden change? Was his high fever a factor?

With regression, typically developing children start to lose their previously acquired abilities. This is most evident in their loss of speech and fine motor skills. Regressive autism usually occurs between the ages of 15 to 30 months. There are some reports that link regression with seizures and some that don't. Cade hasn't experienced seizures since that day. Reports have also linked autism to such things as pollution, pesticides, genetics, parental age, prescriptions taken by the child's mother, vaccines and gluten. Whether or not any of these things cause autism isn't my expertise. I am not a scientist, neurologist or psychologist. I am merely a parent. And as a parent, my job is figuring out the best way to deal with all of this crap.

Drifting gloomily in a cloud of darkness was proving to not be the best way. I had to kick my self-pity aside and focus on my son. There are defining moments in life that shape who we are. The pain, sorrow and loss will either break you or transform you into something more powerful than you'd ever imagined. Committed to making the best life possible for my son, I listened. I listened to a voice that was there all along. You see, parents have a unique ability that's hard to describe. We have intuition.

Our intuition lets us know the difference between a hungry cry and a dirty diaper cry. Silently, my child was crying beneath his monstrous facade and it was time for his voice to be heard.

Many years have passed since then. Observing Cade and the world around us, I still wonder what life would be like without the ability to verbalize my feelings. Communication is such a crucial tool for survival. And although silence is golden, it can be agonizing in our times of need. It's late spring and the tree pollen still covers our vehicles like powdered sugar over beignets.

"Uggh." Cade grunts on the couch.

The sounds of pain and frustration are heard all throughout the night. My Cade radar is on high alert keeping REM sleep at bay.

"God, please grant my son peace." I pray.

Tears cross my lips while tightly gripped my hands remain.

"Please keep him free from pain."

There's no worse feeling than knowing your child is suffering.

"Please..."

At times the man upstairs appears to be listening. Then, there are times when I swear that he must be preoccupied with more pressing matters. Either way, I continued to pray.

6:00 a.m. comes way too soon. My hands still gripping. My heart still praying. I make my way to the living room. Cade has recently decided that he likes sleeping on the couch. That's

Don't Squeeze the Spaceman's Taco

fine with us. After all, Cade is a teenager and teenagers need the freedom to make their own decisions.

"Uggh…" His grunting gets louder.

The heavy wood frame hammers the floor as Cade slams his 250 pound body against the couch. Repeatedly he jerks with the greatest of force. Scrambling, I retrieve his migraine pill. Then, with one last thud the trial is over. That's when the sturdy couch shifts sending our tall mahogany end tables crashing to the floor. Julee's favorite lamps once rested atop these tables. It was during a previous meltdown that we found them shattered across the terracotta tiles.

"Here Cade." I reach out to him. "This will help you feel better."

With water cascading down his shirt, he swallows the pill that I gave him.

"Now," I assure him. "The headache will be gone real soon."

"It's gone real soon!" Throwing the plastic cup across the room he shouts. "It's gone real soon! It's gone real soon! It's gone real soon!"

"Try to relax son."

"It's gone real soon! It's gone real soon! It's gone real soon!" The forceful stomping echoes throughout our house.

"Please try to relax son." I implore. "I'm going to go make your breakfast."

Crossing through the doorway to the kitchen I step over the bits of sheetrock dusted across the floor. Yet another hole in the wall.

"Breakfast is ready buddy."

Cade approaches the dining room table and awaits his breakfast burrito.

"Ooh..." Speaking of himself in the third person he continues. "You broke the TV."

Cade always gives himself away when he's done something bad. Slowly I cross over the dusting of sheetrock and hope for the best. I, of all people, should know better. The television screen is annihilated.

"Why the hell would you do that?" Furiously, I yell as loudly as I can.

Tired of repairing and tired of replacing my rampage endures. Ashamed of what he's done, Cade buries his face into his palms. That's when it hits me. Cade's frustration stems from his chronic pain. My buddy is plagued with limited verbal skills and without a voice to be heard, destruction is inevitable. I recall my father having a stroke when I was growing up. The challenges presented during his recovery remain vivid to this day.

The room was dimly lit. My father's eyes remained sensitive following an ischemic stroke; the type of stroke that's caused from blood clots. Our Louisiana home lacked the usual smell of a southern kitchen. However, with dietary restrictions Mom set out to make the best baked chicken and broccoli possible. My father may have been craving her fried chicken with baked macaroni and mashed potatoes. However, doctor's orders didn't allow it.

"I made your dinner," Mom gently called out to him.

Holding his right forearm, Dad glanced over his dinner plate. With a look of disappointment he reluctantly took a seat. Then gently he lifted his right arm and placed it upon the table.

Mom released the push and seal top of her yellow Tupperware pitcher, and filled my father's glass. Unsweetened iced tea has always been somewhat of an abomination in the south, but you learn to get used to it.

As Dad took his first bite, an unexpected look of gratitude appeared. To my surprise, he actually enjoyed the healthy meal. Not a word was spoken until the very last bite. Then, contently he leaned back into his chair. The smile on his face told me all that he was about to say. A sudden twitch and his head shifted to the side. Opening his mouth, he attempted to speak but sadly there was no sound. Taking a deep breath, he attempted once more. The unwelcomed silence was deafening. I could sense the rage that was building within. Furiously, Dad's left fist pounded the table.

"Casie," Mom called out. "The doctor said not to get worked up. It's bad for your blood pressure."

Unclenching his fist, Dad closed his eyes. His chest rose as he inhaled. Gradually he re-opened his eyes. Glancing towards the love of his life, he parted his lips. Again he attempted to speak. And that's when his frustration reached a boiling point. Swiftly he rose with his right arm falling heavily to his side. My mother's favorite dishes began soaring throughout the room. Although Dad had been right handed all of his life, his left arm was proving to be quite powerful. With a carpenter's grip, he flipped the kitchen table on its side. I ducked as the last of Mom's wheat patterned dinner plates shot above my head.

What was Dad trying to say? What was it that triggered such a destructive outburst? My father eventually regained his speech. Months later, while drinking from the last surviving coffee mug from that evening, I asked him.

"The words were on the tip on my tongue." He replied. "But nothing would come out."

We sat there a moment, Dad and I. Laughing, we gazed over the kitchen cupboard. Mom had just replaced all of our dishes with Tupperware. What was it that he was trying to say that dreadful evening? It was actually something quite simple.

"Thank you."

Staring at the shattered TV screen, I repeat my father's words. "But nothing would come out... But nothing would come out..."

I often think about these words and the power of communication. When Cade is hurting and he can't express his pain, that's when the wreckage begins. When the people in our community are hurting and we ignore their plea, that's when the wreckage begins. There's been a wave of protests and riots erupting across our nation. It all stems from years of political injustice. When people are hurting and they finally have the courage to speak up, the least that we can do is listen. Listen to the voices of those in need. For without a voice to be heard, destruction is inevitable.

"So Cade..." Taking a deep breath, I close my eyes and pause. "What would you like to do today?"

"Dad," speaking of himself in the third person he continues. "You watch *Aladdin*."

"But what will we watch it on?" I ask. "You broke the TV."

"Ooooohhhh...." With his eyes opened wide he sighs and scolds himself. "You broke the TV... No TV for you... No video for you... No *Aladdin* for you, Cade... You broke it."

"How about helping me clean up all this mess, and then we can play *Aladdin*?" I suggest. "I will be the Genie and you can be Aladdin."

And that's the quickest clean up job I've ever witnessed. An hour later and Cade and I are still playing *Aladdin*. It's easy enough though. Cade knows all of the lines. All I have to do is hang around and grant him his wishes.

"Hello boys." Julee announces as she opens the door. "I'm home."

I have to admit, I can do a pretty damn good Iago voice. My Jasmine voice, on the other hand, now that's a different story. In a scene where Iago is imitating Jasmine, I call out to Julee, "Will you come here?"

"What?" Snickering and a bit confused she asks. "Where are you?"

"Ahem…In the menagerie, hurry."

"You are twisted." She exclaims with clear certainty. "And that's why I love you."

Cade and I carry on ignoring Julee. Not to be rude, but we still had a few more scenes left to reenact. It doesn't bother her very much though. She just smiles, puts down her red leather purse and joins us on the living room floor.

"Well, you boys continue playing." She announces after being our understudy for Princess Jasmine. Standing up, she proceeds towards the kitchen. "I'm going to get started on dinner."

Julee loves to cook and Cade loves to eat, so it's shaping up to be a great evening after all.

"*Game of Thrones* comes on tonight," excitedly she announces. "And I really can't miss this one."

"Yeah…" I reply. "About that…"

Staring at the shattered TV screen, I repeat my father's words. "But nothing would come out… But nothing would come out…"

Chapter 12

Cade goes to the Prom

Once upon a time there was a handsome young boy named Cade. He lived with his mother, father and his daring Uncle Brett. Everyone did their very best to keep Cade happy and giggly. Aside from his loving family, Cade also lived with two wicked ailments. Chronic allergies and migraines treated the charming lad badly. One day Cade's teacher left a note in his Batman backpack. It was an invitation to the school prom. Cade was very excited to receive the big news. Merrily, he envisioned himself dancing the night away to DJ Snake and Lil John shouting "Turn Down for What." Joy gleamed from his parents' eyes as they watched their son smile. But lurking in the background were Cade's two wicked ailments. And they would stop at nothing to keep him from having a good time. Allergies and migraines have ruined many of Cade's big days.

As time went on, the week of prom soon arrived. Still counting down the days, Cade boarded a carriage with his parents and off they went. Cade's mom had pressing matters to tend to in a land far, far away. To assist in the journey, Cade and his father transported her to the airport. The company for which Cade's mom worked would be presenting at a convention in Las Vegas, Nevada. Saying farewell, she left for her departing gate. The next several days will be just the boys.

In grand celebratory style, Cade and his father had dinner at one of his favorite eateries. While dining the two conversed on how much they will miss Cade's mother the coming week. Licking his fingers, Cade summoned the lovely young maiden for more chicken wings. Her bosoms lightly brushed against his shoulder. Reaching over, she added to the feast already on the table. Enthusiastically, the two men lifted their glasses.

"Cheers!" They shouted.

Good times were had by all as they laughed, told stories and smacked their chicken bones clean. Adorned in their owl tank tops, the ladies provided exceptional service that afternoon.

With their bellies full, Cade and his father traveled east. The local movie theater promised two hours of non-stop action and explosions. Oddly enough, the pulse pounding adrenaline aided with the digestion of their chicken wings. As the final credits rolled, Cade and his father exited the theater and re-entered their carriage. Tired from a long, busy day they both prepared for a good night's rest.

It was 11:30 a.m. the next morning when Cade finally woke up. Of course there was no point in attending school at such a late hour so Cade would just stay home.

"Whatever will I wear?" Cade wondered.

There were only two days remaining until the prom. And although he had seen photographs of such festive events he had never attended one.

"We must visit the Tuxedo Lady." Cade's father gestured. "For only she can deliver the dapperness."

And so Cade and his father journeyed to the mystical Tuxedo Lady's shop. It was during a previous visit that she collected his precise measurements. Glancing him over, she casted an enchanted spell.

"A one and a two and a wikkity wokkity woo…"

The Tuxedo Lady's magic transformed Cade into a debonair young man. Looking down at his feet, he wiggled his toes.

"Oh my," declared the Tuxedo Lady. "We've got to do something about that…Hmmm…" She deliberated. "Wait! I've got just the right thing… A three and a four, now you're smooth down to the floor."

A pair of shiny new patent leather shoes finished it all off.

Looking in the mirror, Cade was overjoyed. "Bad ass!" He exclaimed edging his fingers across his lapel.

The following daybreak Cade rose from his royal twin bed. Hanging from his bedpost was his beloved custom tuxedo. Breakfast had been prepared and awaited the eager young man in the kitchen.

"Tomorrow is the big day." Cade's father declared.

Without a word, Cade's smile said it all. It was certainly shaping up to be a fantastic day. Fantastic in every way but one, that is. Or should I say two? Cade's wicked ailments threatened to emerge from the darkness. First up was his evil allergies. Dreadfully, they began their torment. In hopes of keeping Cade's nasty migraine at bay, his father worked quickly. He must defeat them before it's too late. Back and forth they clashed. It was an epic battle of good vs evil as Dad took on the bitter adversaries. In a fiery rage, Cade's migraine exploded. Exhausted and beat down, Cade's father persisted. For he would risk everything to ensure his son's happiness. And although they put up a tenacious fight, the vicious ailments were soon defeated. The remainder of the day was back to the usual Cade; happy and giggly.

"Today is the big day!" Excitedly, Cade's father shouted.

It was as if he had scratched off the winning lottery ticket. The morning passed with no sign of Cade's wicked ailments. Perhaps there was a silver lining to yesterday's dark cloud. If there was to be a debilitating headache, it was better to have it yesterday than to have it today. With his hair slicked back, Cade was suited up from head to toe.

"There's something missing." His father proclaimed.

Opening the box held tightly in his hand, he took out a yellow rose. Carefully, he pinned the flower to the lapel of Cade's coat. Then, taking a step back he nodded and affirmed.

"Bad ass, my son! Now off you go to the prom."

Later that day Cade's father received a message from the ruler of his son's school. Principal Howe was a noble leader indeed. In her memo, it was noted that Cade was the life of the party. He and his class mates danced the entire afternoon. The students enjoyed a delicious meal and shared hours of precious laughter. Eagerly awaiting his son's return, Cade's father paced their uphill driveway. Moments later and just a couple blocks away, the stage coach finally came into view. Cade's father waited patiently for the driver to come to a complete stop. Then the screeching doors expanded and there he was, the fresh prince of Belmont. With an enormous grin, Cade stepped down from the vehicle. And yes, he was still wearing both shoes. That shit only happens in fairy tales.

Eager to share the story of our past week, we leave to pick up Julee at the airport. Cade had just gotten home from school and the two of us scan the travelers lining the platform.

"Momma!" Cade shouts.

And there she is with her hair pulled loosely back. She's wearing tortoiseshell sunglasses filtering the glare from the mid-afternoon sky. Cade glances over his mom's rich auburn hair and big gleaming smile to swiftly grab the gift bag that's hanging from her forearm. Excitedly, he rips the bag apart.

"Wolverine! Ahhhh…" He shouts.

Nothing says I care like a bendable action figure of your favorite Marvel superhero and an Elvis Presley t-shirt. Combining the two, Cade transforms himself into the King of Mutants.

"I could sure go for some ice cream." Julee declares as we head back to the house.

Cade sits still smiling. Content with his new toy, he looks down at his shirt.

"Mom," asks Cade. "What kind of ice cream does Elvis like?"

"Elvis," replies Julee. "He likes peanut butter and banana ice cream."

"Yeah," agrees Cade. "Mom," again he asks. "What kind of ice cream does Wolverine like?"

"Wolverine likes chocolate."

"Yeah..."

Cade takes Julee by the hand and together they skip into Ben & Jerry's. Julee honestly looks as if she's going to explode with excitement. It's funny what ice cream does to an adult.

"It's a great day for Chunky Monkey," greets the bubbly young woman from behind the counter.

She has pink wavy hair and arms covered in anime tattoos. It's as if a bored carnival worker stuck her head in the cotton candy machine just for the heck of it. But I like that in a person. She's an unexpected combination of the many flavors in the case before her.

"What do you want?" Cade asks himself while leaning against the chilled glass.

"Let's see... Um..." He replies. "You want Cherry Garcia."

"Yummy." The young woman declares in delight. "That's one of my favorites."

"What's your name?" Cade reaches his hand over the glass case and asks.

"Kathy," she replies.

"Kathy… Hey… Are you happy?"

"Why yes I am happy," she answers. "What's your name? And more importantly, are you happy."

"Yes… Cade… Hey Kathy… You have a dog?"

"I do have a dog."

"What's your dog's name?" He asks.

"Goku," she states with a smile.

"What kind of dog is Goku?"

"Goku is a Shih Tzu."

"Goku is a boy." Cade questions with a statement.

"Goku is a boy," she concurs.

While seated, I overhear the family at the adjacent table. They're a quaint little British family, most proper in every way. I think about us and the way that we make a spectacle everywhere that we go. Even though it's merely an ice cream shop, the well-mannered bunch sit with their elbows off the table and their napkins placed neatly across their laps. No doubt, Mum has ever wrestled across an ice cream parlor table with mint chocolate chip shoved up her nose. I listen, curious to hear the life of a typical family of five.

Mother scrapes her dainty spoon across the edges of her cone. Sitting back, she reminisces on the days of her children's early development. I hear talk of strolling her beloved babies throughout the town shoppes in their canopy covered prams. And how knackered she was having three children so close in age while renovating their countryside estate.

"Mum," prompts the oldest of the three. The young lad appears not far from seven years old. "Remember when I used to suck your tit?"

And just like that I feel as if I'm part of the group – the "normal" group. Apparently children of all backgrounds will figure out a way to embarrass their parents. The look on Mum's face tells me that we're more alike than I initially anticipated.

We leave the ice cream parlor to a very familiar sound.

"Brummmm…."

Brother-in-law Brett zips by on his faithful little scooter. Looking towards me, he shakes his head.

"Ooooh, you dribble drot!"

Then just as quickly as Brett appears, he drifts slowly out of site. The lone wolf, dark and mysterious; he rides alone. Julee, Cade and I get back into my car. I pair my phone and I select some tunes for our ride home.

"Who's that?" Cade queries.

"That's Missy Elliott, buddy."

"Daddy…"

"What buddy?"

"Get Ur Freak On."

"That's right buddy." I confirm. "Get Ur Freak On."

I set my Itunes on repeat and for the next ten minutes we bounce, jump and throw it down with Missy Elliott. Bit by bit I crank the music up louder. By the time we arrive home we're all slightly deafened for a few brief moments. Julee unpacks her suitcase, Cade plays with his new toy and I sit on the back porch thinking.

"Who's going to crank up the music when I'm no longer around?"

I often wonder about things like this. Submerged in worry, I think about the little things that Cade enjoys. Will anyone else go the extra mile to make my buddy's day a little brighter than the day before? Will anyone else keep the traditions that Cade enjoys alive? Nervously, I rock back and forth as I think about these things, especially Cade's favorite traditions.

Traditions--we all have them. Good or bad, they're a part of who we are. Whether it's eating "cock" on Good Friday or dancing a second line at your best friend's wedding, traditions provide comfort. And there's not a more comforting time for traditions than the holiday season.

And if you ask Cade, the official start of the holiday season is Halloween. Our tradition -- carving pumpkins and watching Tim Burton's *The Nightmare Before Christmas*. My job at Halloween is similar to that of a prep cook. I get the pumpkins ready so that Cade can create his masterpiece. Here's how that works.

"Daddy," referring to himself in the third person, Cade continued. "Who you gonna be for Halloween?"

"I don't know buddy. Who are you going to be for Halloween?"

"Fred Flintstone!" He smiled and eagerly awaited as I gutted his pumpkin. The slimy strands oozed between my fingers.

"Daddy..."

"What buddy?"

"Fred Flintstone has dirty feet."

"Yes he does, Cade." My hands deep in pumpkin brains, I chuckled. "Yes he does."

Putting one foot in front of the other, I delivered the artist his canvas. Meticulously he worked. His small utensil furrowed until his sculpting was complete. Two triangle shaped eyes, a triangle shaped nose and a crooked mouth.

"Wow Cade!" I applauded. "Who's that?"

"Bat Man." He proclaimed in a bad ass Caped Crusader voice. "Daddy..."

"What buddy?"

"Make Superman."

Taking my cue, I cleaned the next pumpkin. It was a rather large gourd with chiseled ribbed features, a pumpkin worthy of the Man of Steel. Watching Cade admire his handy work made me smile. It wasn't enough though, to keep my tears from falling. You see, Cade loves carving pumpkins. Who's going to carve pumpkins with him when I'm gone? Lost in infinite worry, I wondered. I wondered what the future held for my son.

One of the hardest things about raising a child with disabilities is the endless worry. With all the things that Cade enjoys, who's going to be there for him when I'm gone? There's so much that he looks forward to this time of year.

"Daddy...October, November, December..."

"Yes Cade...October, November, December..."

"First Halloween," joyfully, he outlined the remainder of the year, "then Thanksgiving, then Christmas."

Ready to take on the man from Krypton, he etched away. Cade remained content in his DC Nation while my mind began to drift. Just like Jack, the Pumpkin King, I thought of the many splendid holidays to come.

The slimy pumpkin strands brought me back to Halloween present. With Cade steadily chipping, Superman was taking form. Two triangle shaped eyes set the stage for things to come. Continuing my clean up the sticky seeds fell to the floor. Excited, Tramp ran over and licked them up.

Humming the Superman theme song his artwork came to life. Two triangle shaped eyes, a triangle shaped nose and a crooked mouth.

"Wow Cade!" Again, I applauded. "That's one cool Superman pumpkin."

"Yeah!" He proudly agreed. "That's one cool Superman pumpkin."

Cade is my best friend. There's not a day that goes by that I don't worry about him. Who's going to worry about him when I'm gone?

Thinking of Cade's favorite traditions, my worries consume me. Back and forth I rock on the patio chairs as dusk begins to fall. It will be at least six more months before Cade and I carve pumpkins again. Gazing out into our back yard, I watch as the tall trees sway. The steady breeze blowing through our wind chimes provides hours of orchestral music. The perfect backdrop for relaxing and instead I'm lost in worry. Feeling myself cave in, I reach out to my mom.

    I recall the times when, just like the trees, Mom swayed to and fro. When struggling to stand tall, she planted her roots firmly on the edge of sanity. As a kid, I remember her emotional battles. I remember how each blow pushed her just a little closer to the brink. I remember when, despite her strength and courage, she fell bitterly into the depths of madness. I remember all the punches and all the blows that mental illness threw at her and yet somehow she managed to climb her way back. I remember how with each fall she collapsed a little bit deeper and with each climb she rose a little bit higher. Mom just never gave up. Instead she grew stronger and instead she grew wiser. Her strength, she said, came from her faith. Mom, in her infinite wisdom, reminds me not to dwell on the worry of tomorrow. But rather, be thankful for the gift of today.

    "Thank You for this Day"

Thank you for this day Dear Lord
My mind will be at peace
I see you as my everything
Your wonders never cease
A song is in my heart today
I see you everywhere
You've given me my life and soul
I needn't have a care
I put my faith in you today
I never need to weep
You're close within my heart today
The bringing of the sheep
How can I count my blessings Lord?
You're always just on time
I see you in the great somewhere
A life just too sublime

Helen Melerine

Slowly my rocking stops as the air becomes still. Missing is the peaceful tinkling of metal rods. I stroll over to the wind chime and slide my finger across the stained glass fleur-de-lis that dangles from its center. The chime has a heavy aluminum frame that beautifully captures the royal colors of the Mardi Gras. On a breezy evening when I'm missing New Orleans, I'll sit on the back patio and listen to the sounds of nature's percussion.

My hand grazes the suspended tubes and I gently close my eyes. Opening them, I turn my head to the side.

"Hello there, Mr. Yang."

The cat stares back at me.

"What do you want cat?"

Yang continues his stare. I think he's happy that the wind finally died down. And yet here I am at damn near ten o'clock creating more annoying racket.

"Shouldn't you be out catching mice?" I muddle.

With no appreciation for my sarcasm, he lifts his rear paw and scratches behind his ear. He then gives me one final glance before wandering off into the night. I go back inside amidst the steady noise of a running vacuum cleaner and Tramp gives me a similar stare.

"What do you want dog?"

With Tramp, it's one of two things. Either he's hungry or he has to crap.

"You hungry?" I ask.

His sudden rapid tail wagging lets me know that I'm on the right track. I reach into the cabinet and pull out a can of his favorite, Kibbles 'n Bits Homestyle. Immediately, Gumbo runs up behind. His warm nose nudges against my butt.

I hook my finger into the pop tab and pull the lid back. The dogs jump up rejoicing in delight and start tap dancing across the kitchen floor. Excitement has built up inside of them and they just can't hide it any longer. I go under the sink, retrieve their bowls, grab a serving spoon from the cutlery drawer and divide the slop unevenly in two. It's only fair that Gumbo gets more than Tramp. He's more than twice Tramp's size. Eyeballing the gourmet guck, I aim to achieve a precise can to dog ratio. Bursting with anticipation, Gumbo does a quick back spin. In all seriousness, he just looks ridiculous dancing to the sound of a droning vacuum cleaner. So I take out my phone and press play to a blast from the past. Tonight the Pointer Sisters will set the mood with "I'm so Excited." Holding their dishes slightly above their heads, I take the lead. When I move forward, they back up. When I mooove to the left, they mooove to the left. We're perfectly in sync with their eyes focused just slightly above their heads.

There's a gentle tap on my shoulder.

"May I cut in?" Julee inquires.

Joining the frenzied fur ball festival, I pass her the smaller bowl. A dance off is under way and we shimmy about the room. How we end up in the family den, I haven't a clue. But the dogs are no longer amused and they dive headfirst into their nightly feast.

"How'd your talk with your mom go?" Asks Julee.

"It was good." Thinking about the elation that Tramp and Gumbo gain from a simple shared can of dog food, I repeat. "It was good."

It appears that the dogs understand Mom's message -- count your blessings and be thankful for the simple things in life.

As Julee and I sit on the floor beside the coffee table, our eyes meet and we smile. Actually, we laugh. The roaring vacuum sound had transformed into a high pitched siren. And that's when we realized that it's actually the chorus to "Crocodile Rock," and Elton John is nowhere to be found. Quietly, we get up and tiptoe towards Brett's room. Oblivious to the opened door, the rock star continues. Unlike giant arenas and football stadiums, Brett's room provides an intimate setting for an entertainer of his magnitude. We stand there upon the red carpet, Julee and I and we enjoy the show.

Brett takes ownership of the stage and works the crowd from every angle. There really isn't a bad seat in the entire house. And although we're watching from backstage, we still have one hell of a view. Brett's tropical print pajama pants are yanked firmly up to his shoulder blades. His considerable butt crack has engulfed a slew of the surfers and coconut trees that are printed on his pajama pants. It's like they're lost somewhere deep within the Bermuda Triangle.

"Get back Gumbo," I mumble. His nose once again nudges against me.

"Woof-woof…"

"Oh hey Gumbo… Hey Julia," Brett acknowledges.

Like a professional, he waited until the song was over. Noticing me standing behind his sister, he acknowledges me as well.

"Hey Tote."

"Hey Brett," I continue. "That was one bad ass performance."

"Yeah Brother," Julee affirms. "That was really good."

"Oh thank you," Brett graciously replies. "You know? It's because I'm such a good singer and I got such a style."

"Yes you do," agrees Julee. "Yes you do."

"So what do you want Tote?" Looking my way, Brett shifts his waistband.

"Nothing Brett." I state with a half-cocked smile. "I just wanted to tell you good night."

"Oh? Good night," he responds. "You depplin drote."

"Good night you dwan dween."

And so we close the door and prepare for bed. Tomorrow is the Special Olympics and our star athlete, Cade is already fast asleep.

The next morning as we prepare for the big games, I think about the ways that we've been programmed to measure success. How do you measure success? Did you get the promotion you've been working so hard to achieve? Is your retirement portfolio sufficient to live the rest of your life comfortably? Perhaps you've met the love of your life. Maybe your children have grown and have lives of their own. Now you're ready to travel the world. Success has many different meanings. Sometime we forget the many great things that we've accomplished in life. Sometime we focus solely on the things that we haven't achieved. Sometime we take for granted that other people's struggles are far greater than our own.

It's an honor to attend the Special Olympics with Cade. The proud moments of accomplishment expressed by the children involved melt my heart. As the athletes line up at their respective starting marks, their eyes remain sharply focused on the finish line. Eagerly, the trained Olympians await their signal. Suddenly, a piercing whistle blows in the background and off they go. And although some run through the finish line, others run around it. Some remain still at the starting mark while others jump joyfully in circles. Victory is not only expressed by the blue ribbon recipients but by every competitor involved. Stations are set up around the field and each athlete does their very best. A feeling of pride is evident throughout the events.

I watch as Cade enjoys his favorite pastime; lunch. The children share a picnic basket filled with their favorite foods. No doubt competing has given them quite an appetite. There are smiles adorning the faces of the many classmates sitting atop their quilted blanket. Smiles on all the kids but one, that is. A beautiful young girl shifts uncomfortably in her seat. Her long brown hair sways as she wriggles side to side. Her magnificent amber eyes fill with tears as she moans in isolation.

"What is she thinking?" I wonder to myself. "What would I do if trapped in a body that I could not control?"

I think for a moment as I approach to greet the lovely young athlete. Not knowing where to start, I just start.

"Do you believe that the Jonas Brothers split up?"

Rambling on a subject that I know so little about, I perform a Google search on my phone. Does she even like boy bands? She could very well be a rock fan or maybe even a country girl. I have no idea. Regardless, I use my newly gained knowledge of Kevin, Joe and Nick and I ramble away. Then, with a twitching movement her hand slowly wipes across her mouth. She stares for a moment then gradually lifts a slice of pizza from her lap. Grease marks tinge the plate from which it lay. Her splendidly crooked smile parts and she nibbles at the crust. While our encounter is brief, it leaves a lasting impression.

The Special Olympics proves to be a great day for Cade. He wins first place in the tennis ball throw event. His sense of happiness and pride is evident as we leave the field. And of course it's a proud moment for me as well. I'm his dad. Regardless, I can't help but think about the girl with the big brown eyes.

"What if she hates boy bands?" I ask myself. "What if she hates boy bands and pizza?"

Imagine a world where we have no choices. A world where someone else makes all of our decisions for us.

The bells clatter as I push the door open.

"Welcome to You'll Take What I Give You and Like it Diner. Have a seat wherever ya like," the waitress shouts peeking through the top of her dark crimson framed glasses. Margie is her name. "No… On second thought, have a seat right over here."

Heeding Margie's instruction, I advance towards an empty booth. The cracked vinyl covering scratches my leg as I scoot along the bright red cushion. I press my elbows against the metal blinds and glance over the menu. Breakfast on one side, lunch and dinner on the other.

"I'll have the bacon cheeseburger and a root beer."

Although I normally make healthy decisions, it's a cheat day. With an undeniable sense of guilt, I place my order. Eagerly waiting, I tap my feet to the oldies but goodies echoing from the jukebox. A little Smokey Robinson and the time zips on by. Soon I'll be feasting on fat and carbohydrates. Finishing six weeks of nothing but grilled chicken and broccoli, the anticipation is killing me. After all, this place was voted the best burger in town four years in a row.

Abruptly, the kitchen door swings open. Margie stands there a moment adjusting her apron. Carrying the goods, she approaches my booth in the adjacent corner. I've been waiting six long weeks to bite into that burger. Just like Pavlov's eager dog, I'm salivating before the plate even touches the table.

"Grits and whole wheat toast," declares Margie as she struts her way out of sight. "Bon appetite."

Life can be very challenging but I am thankful for the ability to make my own decisions. My heart aches for the many things that my son may never experience -- like going to college or falling in love. However, I am thankful for the many great things that I know he will achieve.

So how do you measure success? To me, it depends on the challenge. Hearing your teenage son or daughter use complete sentences may not excite most parents. But to me, it's worthy of a blue ribbon. Success in raising a child with disabilities is best measured by smaller accomplishments. There are days that can be very dark. It's in the darkness that it's best to look back and realize just how far you've come.

I hope one day, following your youngest child's wedding, you find yourself traveling the world with the love of your life. I hope this elaborate trip is paid for with only a small piece of your investment portfolio. I hope one day, while relaxing on the shores of Fiji, exploring the pyramids of Egypt or safariing through Africa, you get a call from your boss. You've just received the promotion that you've been working towards your entire life. I hope one day, when this new job brings you stress, you can lay back, prop your feet up on your desk and smile. You recall the day that you informed that asshole from accounting that you're his new boss.

Chapter 13

Summertime with Nana

> I love my Nana the most
> Nana the most
> Nana the most
> I love my Nana the most
> Yes I do

"Nana" is what Cade calls my sister Iris. Yes, she taught him this song. Yes, he sings it at the top of his lungs. Yes, he means every word of it. Do you have a Nana? Perhaps it's an aunt or uncle, a teacher, that special friend or mentor. The person that always believed in you. The one that held your hand as you dissected your way through life. What if you had a chance to repay this person? What would you do?

It's shortly following Memorial Day, an unusually hot morning as I prepare for work. Exhausted, Julee and I stare in the bathroom mirror. With matching dark circles, our eyes tell a story.

"How's my hair?" I query.

It was a rough night but never underestimate the power of good hair. Slowly Julee's eyes drift over.

"Really?" She questions. "Are you really worried about your hair right now?"

"Somebody got up on the wrong side of the bed." With a smack on her bottom and a kiss on her cheek I continue, "If only we were lucky enough to go to bed last night."

Don't Squeeze the Spaceman's Taco

Cade's allergies spawned a tornado of a migraine that ravaged our happy home. By 4:00am we picked up the shattered glass and sighed. Cade was finally calm and fast asleep on the couch. Worried that we would get no sleep the next couple hours, we got no sleep.

Raising a child with disabilities is both physically and financially draining. There are seasons of darkness that will challenge your very core. Fortunately, a beacon of hope approaches on the horizon. Summertime with Nana is something that Cade longs for autumn through spring. Nana's a small framed woman with a big heart. Growing up, she was always the backbone of my family. With fifteen years between us she has been my sister, friend and mentor for as long as I can remember. Iris and I share the same pointy nose and chin, the same brown eyes and the same brown curly hair. We're both prone to frizziness in the southern humidity. So just like me, she appreciates a good hair day.

She was always a generous soul, my sister. Her own financial burdens didn't matter. Perhaps she got that from my grandmother. Mémère Mary lived a very meager life. What little she did have she gave away. Even on the coldest winter days, her sincere goodness warmed my heart.

There was an Arctic blast approaching the bayou. At times, the most southern parts of Louisiana can become bone-chilling. With several space heaters going, Mémère Mary did what she could to keep her modest trailer warm. Concerned for her comfort, I went shopping for the heaviest quilt that I could find. I was just fifteen years old at the time. With money that I saved by working on a shrimp boat I purchased the quilt. My grandmother lived alone once my grandfather passed. Alone until someone needed help, that is. Her door was always open to those in need. At the time, my brother Casie was living with her. Casie was in his thirties. Suffering from mental illness, he rarely kept a job.

Proud of the deal that I got on the quilt, I called my grandmother.

"I just wanted to make sure that you were home. I'd like to stop by for a visit."

"Come on over baby. I'll be waiting for you."

And waiting she did. Mémère Mary paced back and forth along the gravel road. To keep warm she was wearing her old faithful house dress, two pairs of socks, fuzzy slippers and a big puffy nylon coat. Being a hand me down from her sister-in-law, the coat was a wee bit snug. The tight squeeze, however, provided extra warmth on such a brisk winter day.

It was around 2:30 in the afternoon when my car turned down the road leading towards her home. Mémère's eyes lit up the way that they always did when she saw me. The lightest shade of blue they were and clear; clear as the sky above. She had the usual Bugler hand rolled cigarette hanging form the corner of her mouth. Smoke rose from the tiny nub, gliding through the fine lines just above her lip.

Passing beside her, I rolled my window down. "Get in and I'll take you back to your house."

"No thank you baby," she insisted. "I'll just walk."

My grandmother had a profound phobia of vehicles. Several years back, she and my grandfather were involved in an automobile accident. While crossing an intersection, a passing vehicle failed to yield and struck their car from the side. Spinning into oncoming traffic, my grandmother held on for dear life. Although no one was injured in the accident, Mémère Mary was never the same. From that moment on, every time that she exited a vehicle she stopped to give Him praise.

"Thank you Jesus!" She'd shout while bending over to kiss the ground.

My grandmother was sixty-five years old and as long as I could remember, she always looked the same. It wasn't that she looked young for sixty-five. But more like she looked sixty-five for the past fifteen years. "Chatty," is how most people described her. "She's never met a stranger," they'd say. Just ask the random man at the hospital who showed her and my family the scars from his recent open-heart surgery; just five minutes after my grandmother introduced herself. Or the clerk at the Godiva Chocolates counter that she lectured on the history of the Rockefeller family. It all started with the simple question, "How much for the chocolate covered cherries?" Appalled by the price of the so-called premium fine chocolates, Mémère contended, "But I am not Mrs. Rockefeller." Or perhaps the young movie usher who learned that the modern cinemas could never possibly compare to the majestic Saenger Theater.

It was during my Christmas break from St. Bernard Community College. Thinking that it would be nice to take my grandmother to see a new movie, we entered the auditorium.

"It's dark in here, Baby!"

"Shhhh…," gesturing to her, I placed my finger against my mouth. "The movie has already started."

"What kind of movie you trying to take me to anyway?"

"It's called *Driving Miss. Daisy*. It's about a cranky old woman and the kind, caring gentleman that has to drive her crotchety old butt around town." Tugging lightly on her arm, I continued. "Look here's a couple seats."

"But I can't see anything," she reiterated. "Why it's gotta be so dark in here? The Seanger Theater was never this dark."

Taking her seat, she finally noticed the movie that was playing. "Well, would you look at that? That sure is a big ole screen?"

I nodded my head in acknowledgement.

"Do you know the Saenger had lights that looked like the stars?" Visualizing the old historic theater, she lifted her hands. "The ceiling looked just like the nighttime sky."

Tugging again at her arm, I leaned over towards her. "The people behind us can't see when you lift your arms up."

"There were clouds that drifted across the sky." Swaying with the movement of the clouds, her hands rose higher. "Oh the Saenger was such a beautiful Theater."

"Yes," I agreed. "And it still is. But you're blocking everyone's view when you lift your arms up like that."

Resting her hands softly on her lap, she enjoyed the next fifteen minutes of the film. As she patted her chest, I knew exactly what was coming next. Removing the roll your own tobacco pouch from her bra, she swiftly lit one up.

"You can't smoke in here Mémère," I informed her.

"But you could smoke in the Saenger Theater."

"Well that was a long time ago."

"Oh for heaven's sake. The last movie I saw was at the Saenger and you could smoke all that you wanted."

The Saenger Theater is a performing arts center in downtown New Orleans and it had been quite a while since movies were shown there.

"When was the last time you went to the movies?" I asked.

"It wasn't that long ago." She pondered for a bit. "Let's see...it was 1952. Your Pépère Robbie took me to see *Singin' in the Rain*. That was such a good movie. Did you see that movie?"

"No. I didn't see it. Well, I've seen parts of it on TV. But things have changed since 1952."

"You can say that again," passing a tiny little granny fart, she continued. "That Gene Kelly sure could dance. And boy was he a good looking man."

Humming the title song to the classic musical, she slouched in her seat. And while the humming was a bit distracting, she did manage to keep it low. Before long I envisioned Morgan Freeman and Jessica Tandy dancing merrily in the street with matching umbrellas. Periodically, I glanced my grandmother's way. Aside from her noticeable nicotine craving, I could tell that she was really enjoying the film. There was a tear in her eye as the aging Daisy Werthan declared Hoke Colburn her best friend. A special moment in film transcended into a special moment in life. As Mémère Mary rose to her feet, her leftover cabbage went to work. The thunderous sound escaping her rear end was reminiscent of a Sunday afternoon monster truck rally.

Pinching my nose I asked, "Where are you going?"

"This is a lovely story Baby, but I gotta find someplace to smoke my cigarette."

Driving Miss Daisy truly was a lovely story. However, Mémère Mary never did return back to her seat. As I exited the theater, I observed her in her usual form. While engaged in conversation, she learned that the teenage movie usher was actually my fourth cousin on my dad's side of the family. And the young man also learned something in return. He learned that regardless of any fancy big screens, the present-day cinemas will never compare to the beloved Saenger Theater.

It was a couple days into the freeze when I called to check on Mémère and Casie.

"Are you keeping warm?" I asked

"Yes baby," she replied. "We're both staying nice and warm. We just have to wear a sweater during the day."

"And at night?" I asked.

"Night time hasn't been bad at all. Thank you so much for the nice quilt that you bought me. I took my scissors and cut it down the middle. Now Casie can sleep well too."

Just like our sharp-cornered facial features and frizzy brown hair, generosity runs deep in my family. From new clothes and school supplies to the latest Prince cassette, whenever in need my sister was always there. She and my brother-in-law SJ gave hope to my teenage years. Aside from shrimp season I spent most of my summer at their house.

Now, some thirty years later, their home has also become a haven for my son to get away. Cade loves summertime with Nana. He loves chatting about Batman on long walks through wooded acres with SJ. Cade calls him Pee-Paw. He loves sharing popcorn at the cinema while watching the latest summer blockbusters with Nana. Cade likes his buttered. He loves dancing while preparing for his upcoming talent show at Camp Sunshine. Cade loves Camp Sunshine -- a week-long celebration for individuals with disabilities. Cade loves the peace and joy of being himself. He loves everything about summertime with Nana, but most of all Cade loves Nana's meatloaf.

Nana stands at the kitchen sink enjoying her first cup of coffee. Peering through the window ahead she smiles. There are two baby deer playing in her back yard. Watching the animals gather is the thing that she enjoys most about living in the country. To attract the gentle creatures, she had a deer feeder installed on her property. She makes sure that the feeder is generously loaded with grain at all times.

"Nana," Cade shouts as he enters the room. "You don't color the man's face gray...," pausing, he waits her reply. "He is not Batman."

"No Cade," she replies. "He is not Batman."

Cade's interactions with my sister always start this same way. He then follows with a series of questions that he specifically designed for her. It's just part of being Cade.

"Breakfast Nana," he requests.

Nana makes the best breakfast. Of course, Nana makes the best everything. Cade knows that during the summer months, whatever precedes the word "Nana" is his for the taking.

"Breakfast Nana..."

"Lunch Nana..."

"Movies Nana..."

"Dollar General Nana..."

My sister never got out much since moving to the middle of nowhere. However, during the summer months, Cade keeps her on the go. Whatever Cade wishes, Nana makes happen. She's like the big blue genie from his favorite Disney movie.

It's a typical Wednesday morning and Cade has asked for breakfast. Putting down her coffee cup, Nana goes straight to work. The first thing in the pan is a pat of butter. If you ask Nana, everything starts with a pat of butter. Soon after, the Holy Trinity fills the air. At the heart of all Creole and Cajun dishes lies the Holy Trinity of spices; a precise blend of onion, celery and bell pepper. Cade steps closer as Nana opens the oven. The warm air brushes across his face. Hypnotically Cade stands by gazing at the made from scratch goodness. Soon Cade is faced with a dilemma. He can either wait for breakfast to be done or just give in now to the fluffy golden layers of Nana's homemade biscuits.

And of course, the biscuits win. Cade just loves a good biscuit. While delivering his plate to the table, Nana smiles. Nana always smiles when preparing Cade's meals. For she knows the elation that Cade has in eating her food. And that type of joy brings her even greater joy.

"What would you like to do today?" She asks.

"Go walking Nana."

It's the third week in July and opening the patio door is like opening the oven door.

"Why don't we wait for Pee-Paw to get home to go walking?"

"Wait for Pee-Paw," Cade repeats.

Pee-Paw always arrives home from work at the optimal walking time. It's during the early evening hours when the sun's not beating down like a beauty salon hairdryer. That's the best time for Cade's long, fast-paced walks. However, if they wait too late, the mosquitos will be out on their nightly hunt. And unfortunately for Cade; mosquitoes love biscuit eaters.

Don't Squeeze the Spaceman's Taco

Avoiding outside activities when it's damn near 100 degrees is always a wise choice. However, Nana is certainly not the kind to just brush Cade off.

"How about we go visit Maw-Maw Helen and Paw-Paw Casie?" She suggests.

"And Uncle Darrin… and Uncle Larry… and Aunt Tina," Cade adds. "And Mr. Willie."

"Yes," agrees Nana. "And Mr. Willie too."

It's a little over 100 miles to our old hometown of St. Bernard Parish. Along the way they stop at the local farmers market. Cade loves the farmers market. He calls it Agrabah, a make believe city in the desert from his favorite movie, *Aladdin*. Agrabah is ruled by the Sultan and home to the royal palace and the Cave of Wonders. In a scene from the movie, the young hero, Aladdin and his monkey companion, Abu scavenge through the marketplace searching for food. The two of them get caught and end up on the run from the palace guards. Cade reenacts this scene by "stealing" apples from the market. Fortunately, Cade knows that if you really do steal you go to jail and if you go to jail you might drop the soap. Therefore, his stealing consists of taking the apples to the cashier and placing one of them in his pocket as he leaves. While paying for their "stolen" goods, Cade picks out a fresh bouquet of flowers for his grandma. Maw-Maw Helen always did love gladiolas.

They arrive for their visit and Cade stands out front. He's holding a vibrant bouquet of flowers in one hand and an apple in the other. Unselfishly he hands over both.

"You go to the market," Cade smiles with his eyes shifting up towards his Nana.

"Tell your grandma all about our trip to the market," Nana suggests.

"You go to the market," Cade repeats excitedly. "You steal the apple. You get flowers. You make poo."

Cade was never one for leaving out details and today he was feeling extra chatty. Fortunately, Maw-Maw Helen was always a good listener. And for the next fifteen minutes Cade elaborates on his trip to Agrabah. It's a great gift to have -- the imagination of a child. Through fantasy Cade can be a commoner turned prince, a superhero in search of justice or anything else that his heart desires. It's sad when we as adults lose this magnificent gift.

Cade raises his eyebrow and looks back towards his grandma.

"Maw-Maw Helen," he queries. "What movies do you like to watch?"

Much like his great grandma Mary, Maw-Maw Helen hasn't been to the movies in many years. In fact, the last time that she has been to the movies was before Cade was born.

"Maw-Maw Helen," Cade replies to himself in the third person. "You like Batman."

"Maw-Maw Helen," again Cade queries. "You have a dog?"

Cade goes through his usual series of questions while Nana cuts the bottom stems from the flowers that they just purchased. Carefully she snips, cutting each one at an angle.

"They last longer this way," she softly whispers.

"Ahem…" Clearing her throat, she hands Cade a tall vase. "Would you go fill this with water for me?"

"They're beautiful." Delightedly, Nana looks over the colorful blossoms. "Although, they're not as beautiful as the ones that you used to grow." With a slight chuckle Nana recalls, "I remember how mad you got when Daddy ran over your flowers with the lawnmower."

There was a narrow strip of grass on the side of my childhood home. The three foot alley ran right alongside Vivian's driveway. This is the place where Mom planted her rosebushes and assortment of flowering annuals. "A flower is God's smile upon us," she would say. "He weeps through his raindrops and then He smiles through his blooms."

Dad, on the other hand, was never concerned with flowers. Monkeyshines is what he called them. Anything not used for practical purposes, my father referred to as monkeyshines. Now Dad did plant numerous fruit trees which he tended to quite regularly and that was perfectly understandable. For each fruit tree had a purpose. They provided a harvest that was edible. And while technically gladiolas are edible, according to my father they were merely monkeyshines. And when it comes to monkeyshines, it's much easier to just plow through them than it is to cut around them.

"Yoo-hoo!" A friendly face leaned in through our front door.

"Come on in Vivian," Mom insisted.

"Girl I was outside washing my car and I said to myself, 'Something seems different.' That's when I noticed your beautiful gladiolas were gone. Why'd you cut them down?" Vivian asked. "They were so pretty and colorful."

"That son of a bitch!" Mom declared as she turned off the gas burner. "Oh, he wants jambalaya, does he? Let him cook it himself."

"Uh-oh." Realizing that she just spilled the beans, Vivian placed her hand over her mouth. "I'm so sorry Helen."

"Don't be sorry for me," Mom asserted. "Be sorry for him when he looks in that pot tonight."

Uncontrollably, Vivian started laughing. "Oh Helen, I'm sorry. I don't mean to laugh but I'm just picturing Casie looking into that empty pot."

Mom's frustration quickly vanished as she too burst with laughter. "I was just about to make a pot of coffee. Why don't you join me?"

"That sounds great," regaining her composure, Vivian continued. "Now there might be nothing in that pot, but whatever's in the oven sure smells good."

Meanwhile, I was lying in bed and life was good. For I knew exactly what Mom had in the oven. It was more of her homemade bread. The loaf that she made earlier was already half gone and stashed away in my bedroom. Melted butter rolled down the corner of my mouth as I indulged.

"Mom said son of a bitch," I snickered in between bites.

My mom never swore but cut down her flowers and the only thing served in her kitchen was revenge. A half coffee pot later and Mom forgot why she was mad in the first place. Friends do that. They make you smile even in your angriest moments. Warm bread and butter, a cup of coffee and laughter with a friend; suddenly gladiola mulch doesn't really matter anymore.

Nana stands there, carefully placing each flowered spike. "Did you know that gladiolas are from the iris family?" She softly questions my mother. "Perhaps that's why you like them so much."

Nana continues arranging the flowers until their just so. A perfectionist, my sister is. It's an honor that I'm the only one that she asks to assist with her household projects. She's always told me that, "If I ask SJ to help, it looks like a toddler did it." Let's just say that my brother-in-law is not as detailed when it comes to home improvement. Stepping back, my sister eyes her arrangement of flowers.

"There, now they look lovely."

Pleased with her work, Nana sits outside on the concrete step. Her head leans against Mom as she watches Cade run through the lush green landscape. It's a peaceful place where my parents are now. It's just a few miles down the road from where we grew up. They're surrounded by friends and family and right across Bayou Road from St. Bernard Catholic Church.

It's always hard for my sister to say good-bye.

"I'm sorry I can't visit as often as I used to," she sadly tells Mom. "Tell Daddy that I love him. Maybe one day we'll move back a little closer."

Blowing my mom a kiss, Nana and Cade walk back to the car. She rolls down her window and the two of them wave good-bye. It's over 100 miles back to Osyka, MS and there's still a few more stops to be made.

The sun hasn't quite begun to set as they head out across Lake Pontchartrain. With any luck, they'll be home in time for Cade's nightly walk with Pee-Paw. Before the mosquitos get too bad, that is. The hot air brushes through Cade's thick golden brown hair as he sticks his head out of the window.

"You're just like your father," Nana tells him. "… Speak of the devil…"

The phone rings and Nana picks it up. "We're on the Causeway Bridge so I'll probably lose the call… Anyway, you'll never guess what Cade is doing."

"What's that?"

"He's hanging his head out the car window looking over the lake – Just like you did when we would go visit Mom in Mandeville."

"That's my boy!" Proudly I exclaim. "I remember that like it was yesterday."

Oddly enough, what seems like yesterday was over thirty-five years ago. No longer synonymous with mental health, Mandeville is now a thriving community. The traffic on the north shore of Lake Pontchartrain reached an all-time peak following Hurricane Katrina. Suddenly uprooted from their community, St. Bernard Parish residents were forced to find new homes. And while some were only temporary, many became permanent. The forty miles stretching from east to west along the northern side of the lake had suddenly changed. A new spice had been added to their gumbo. And all I can say is, "Thank God for GPS." You see, on the north shore, there are no such directions as 'up the road' and 'down the road.'

Sure enough, ten minutes into our conversation I lose my sister's call. Later, while talking to my mom I remember to give thanks. I thank Mom for all that she's done for me throughout the years and for all that she continues to do. I also remember to thank God. I thank Him for giving me my rather unusual family. I thank Him for the strength to keep going and for the wisdom gathered along the way. I especially give thanks for my sister. Without her, I wouldn't know what to do. Before saying good night, Mom had this to share with me.

"Queen of Heaven"

Oh Mother Mary, queen and love
Come light and love divine
Horizons in the sunset true
Embrace this heart of mine
Oh mother of the universe
The roses heaven sent
The brightest morning glories too
Your love is what they meant
Enkindle Holy Spirit true
Oh lady lovely fair
I look unto a bright new day
And know that you are there
I sing unto the canticle
The music of delight
Thine eyes have seen the glory, Lord
Abounding in thy sight

Helen Melerine

    To this day, my sister remains the glue that binds my side of the family together. Because of her, Cade has a stronger relationship with his grandparents, his Uncle Darrin, Uncle Larry, Aunt Tina and Mr. Willie too. The love and guidance received from her and my brother-in-law are irreplaceable. So, how do you repay people like them? You repay them through growth. You repay them by becoming a better person. Much of who I am today, I owe to their love and support. The best way to repay the Nana in your life is to live. Live life for the precious gift that it is knowing that one day our summertime will be over.

Chapter 14

Dance

Julee and I sit side by side in front of our computer. It all looks so perfect. At least Travelocity makes it seem that way.

"They should create a website for families like ours," I suggest while clicking through the idyllic images. "You know? A site that shows pictures of everyone stressed out and ready to go home."

While charting a course for our next adventure, we recall the lessons learned from vacations past.

It was day one of our last family vacation and things were getting off to a rather bumpy start.

"Why bother?" Staring in the bathroom mirror, I asked myself. "Why bother attempting a family vacation?"

The scratches across my forehead and neck gave me second thoughts. Traveling with autism presents many unique challenges. I glanced at the time on my phone. It was a quarter past ten in the morning and we should have been on the road several hours ago. I then glanced up at the newly framed photo sitting atop our bathroom shelf. Tapping on the glass I smiled. My friend, Leidy took Cade to a very special dance. Tim Tebow's Night to Shine Prom is an event like no other. The event provides a magical prom night experience for individuals with special needs ages 14 and older. The smile on Cade's face evidenced the sheer joy of the evening.

Turning back towards the mirror, my skin was gruesomely pale. My eyes still red and swollen. I dabbed antibiotic cream across my neck. Again I glanced at the time on my phone.

"We should have been on the road." I told myself.

Luckily we weren't. Our earlier attempt didn't end so well.

"What should we do about breakfast?" Julee asked.

"Let's just pick up drive through along the way." I replied. "It will save us some time."

Moments later Cade reached into the brown paper bag. Taco Bell was what he wanted and Taco Bell was what he got.

"When you going to Uncle Darrin's house?" Cade questioned himself in the third person.

When Cade asks this question it's a clue that a migraine is on the way. It was an unusually warm winter. Therefore, February had an unusually high pollen count. Unfortunately, Cade's migraines are triggered by allergies. And before long, he was reaching for the hood of my sweatshirt. With my neck pulled back I swerved upon the steering wheel.

"Calm down!" I yelled as Julee gave Cade his pain reliever.

Breakfast tacos and Fire Border sauce exploded inside our squeaky clean rental car. Reading the packet stuck to my side window, I rolled my eyes…"I spontaneously bust out in Ninja moves." My fortune came to me in the form of packaged picante sauce. Abruptly my head jerked to the left. Struggling to keep my eye on the road, I pulled away. A fistful of hair fell to my shoulder. Determined to get home safely, I prayed. The hood of my sweatshirt made for an easy target. Again Cade pulled me back. Julee did her best to keep him down, but with one hand on my neck and the other on my forehead, his nails dug in deeper.

"Calm down!" Again I yelled.

Julee continued holding Cade back and at this point Brett became frightened.

"I'm going to jump out!" Brett cried. "I'm going to jump out!"

"Brett," I continued, "I need you to keep calm as well."

"But I don't want to get in a wreck." In anguish, he screamed.

"We're almost home, Brett."

Once more the hood of my sweatshirt was within Cade's grasp. As he pulled back, the slider of my jacket's zipper pierced the skin on my neck. The more Cade pulled, the more the zipper cut.

"Calm down!"

With both hands upon the steering wheel, I miraculously drove us home. Julee prepared Cade's warm bath and inside the guest bathroom, I tended to my wounds.

"Why bother?" I kept questioning myself. "Maybe we should just stay home."

Putting away the tube of Neosporin, I glanced at the photo from Cade's dance. Again it made me smile. For I knew exactly why we needed a family vacation. And it was a lesson I learned from a complete stranger. It's no coincidence that this stranger and I met. God places people in our lives when we need them most. Although no words were exchanged, this brief encounter changed my life forever.

It was the night of a fraternity party held in the historic Garden District of New Orleans. Creole tunes echoed as we strolled along St. Charles Avenue. The hanging moss flitted as the brisk air drifted down the road. It was winter in the Big Easy. Not terribly cold, but just right for a sweater. At thirty-three years old I was a new pledge in a social fraternity. Don't ask me how that happened. It just did. Down on life after accepting that my son had a life-long disability, I returned to school. My young friend Chris became my big brother and I pledged TKE

"Don't drink too much big bro." In my usual overprotective manner, I went on. "But if you do and I am already gone, please call me."

"You bet lil bro."

As we walked towards the building a woman caught my eye. It's not unusual for a woman to garner attention in this city. New Orleans ladies possess a beauty that is unrivaled. Many chart topping songs have been written about this very phenomenon. Still, there was something uniquely different about this one. Bundled near a trash can, she sang a happy tune. With her face planted into the ground, she continued humming as we walked on by.

While the air may have been warmer inside the bar, the music certainly wasn't. Unbuttoning my sweater, I ordered a round of cocktails. I don't usually drink, but when I do I'm a vodka man. The speakers were pumping and the pussies were popping. Big booties shook as the bitches got low. My, how song lyrics have changed throughout the years. And even though 50 Cent insisted that it was my birthday, I was feeling exceptionally blue.

A slight chill brought my attention towards the doorway and there she was. The homeless lady from the street had just wandered into the bar. Removing her torn coat, the catchy hook from "In Da Club" called her to the dance floor. I pushed my glass aside and watched in amazement. There I was whining about my problems, yet this incredible woman found a reason to dance. Less than ten minutes later she was gone and my outlook on life was changed.

Amid the chaos in life, there is always a reason to dance. A family vacation provides many great memories for years to come. And being the parent of a child with disabilities, you learn to let the good memories overshadow the bad.

Sitting at the computer, Julee and I scan through our own vacation images. Ironically, our photos are very similar to the ones that we see on the travel sites. These are the memories that we choose to keep. Years from now, while looking back upon this disastrous trip, we will not dwell on the afternoon that Cade gave me matching scratches along the back side of my neck. Nor will we occupy our minds with the evening that he vomited across the table in the fine dining room. And we will especially block out Cade eating his vomit while we tried to discreetly clean it all up. So what was brother-in-law Brett doing through all of this? The usual. Brett was worrying about Brett. Moving his plate to the side to avoid contact with the vomit, Brett finished his main course and was asking for dessert. Overall, it was an amazing trip. There were special moments from this trip that we will cherish forever.

We remain giddy, the two of us laughing about the moments not captured on film. All is lighthearted. That is, until my phone rings.

"It's Pookie!" Excitedly I answer. "Hey brother. What's up?"

"I have bad news…"

Nothing good ever starts with these four words. The next three are even harder.

"I have cancer."

Paralyzed in emotion, I hang on to every word. Each uttered syllable is like watching him step across a tightrope. My heart races as he courageously treks forward. Empathetically, I envision myself walking behind him.

"Don't look down," I tell myself. "Stay positive for Pookie."

"They discovered cancer cells during my hernia surgery." He informs me.

"Don't look down," I remind myself.

"But you told me the hernia surgery was a success."

"It was," he matter-of-factly responds. "No more hernia troubles."

I listen as he bravely continues. My palms sweat with each suspended movement as if he's a thousand feet in the air.

"It turns out that I have colon cancer…" He tells me. "Stage IV."

And that's the moment that I look down. Suddenly I'm frozen in grief. I relive the day that Pookie and I met in math class; the day that a tap on the shoulder changed my life forever. "What's the answer to number 3?" was the question that he asked.

Still processing the announcement of Pookie's terminal illness I articulate, "Twenty-five."

"Come again?" He questions me. "Maybe I'm just loopy from the pain medicine, but what did you just say?"

"Twenty-five," I repeat.

"Ok...," again he seeks clarification. "Twenty-five what?"

"The answer to number 3 is C," with profound certainty I continue. "Twenty-five."

Many great memories flash before me and that's when I realize something important. I realize how foolish it is to miss someone who is still here.

"I'm on my way to Austin." I inform him.

"When are you coming?" He asks.

"I can leave tomorrow." Changing my search parameters, I continue, "I was already online looking up travel shit."

"Why don't you wait a few weeks?" He insists. "I have a colectomy coming up."

"When is it?" I ask. "I can be there with you."

"No," again he insists. "Give me some time to recover. I'd rather show you around the city than show you around the hospital. Bring one of your friends with you just in case I can't keep up."

Three weeks later, my friend Mike and I board a plane to Austin, TX; a city that encourages folks to keep it weird. We arrive at Pookie's house traveling with class – economy class. Pulling into his driveway, I honk slightly on the horn. A familiar face whips the striped curtains open and gestures, "One moment."

"Boy what took your ass so long to get here?" Pookie's head peeps out of the screen door exiting his house. "The airport ain't that far from here."

Other than being exceptionally slim, Pookie looked really good. His usual sarcastic manner let me know that he was in good spirits.

"You know," I tell him. "You look a lot like Barack Obama now that you dropped some weight."

"Some weight? How about forty pounds."

"Hey I'm Mike by the way." My friend announces from the back seat. "I've heard a lot about you." Leaning his head to the side Mike continues, "You really do look like Barack Obama."

"I'm Marcel," he gives his fingers a quick snap. "And I approve this message."

Pookie pulls the visor down and glances into the mirror. Rubbing his fingers along his frail jawline, his eyes shift towards Mike's reflection.

"You can call me Pookie."

"So where are we going?" I ask.

"Well you're in Texas and it's breakfast time." Grinning, he flips the visor back up. "Let's do what Texans do and go get a burrito. There's a place near the prison where I work that's really good."

Pookie tunes the radio as we drive off into town. He and Mike sing along to nearly every song that's playing. Remaining quiet, I tap my fingers to the music. Let's just say that singing is not my thing. It takes roughly fifteen minutes for me to drive to the crowded little shack. But if you ask Pookie, it should have only taken me twelve. The graveled parking lot is full. Why so many people pack into a burrito joint at 9:30 am on a weekday morning is beyond logic to me. It must be some damn good burritos is the only rational explanation. I circle the lot a couple times in search of an available spot. Seven young men suddenly cram into a light blue Ford Pinto and they leave. In sync, Pookie and I crack up.

"Reminders of the good old days," he sneers.

We recall piling into Pookie's first car, a Ford Pinto nonetheless. It was the same pastel shade of blue – a color you'd expect to find in a dollar store eye shadow. We were just a group of kids from down the road exploring the big city of New Orleans. "Laissez les bon temps rouler?" Indeed we did.

"At least they didn't have to push start their car." Laughing hysterically, I lean forward and gas erupts from my butt.

"Good Lord boy!" Pookie opens the door and jumps out. "You done shit on yourself?"

We cover a lot of ground by mid-afternoon. Roaming through town, Mike and Pookie continue belting out melodies. My economy car was living up to Austin's nickname of the live music capital of the world. As for me, let's just say that my finger tapping improves and bit by bit I hum along.

"I'm getting a little hungry," I announce.

A few miles down the highway and Pookie directs me to an exit. "Turn here," he declares. "This is my favorite spot."

"If this is another burrito joint, I do not object," I tell him. "Breakfast was delicious."

"No," he assures me. "This is way better than a burrito joint."

By the time we stop my rental car feels like a four cylinder karaoke bar. Pookie exits and we follow swiftly behind. Dust settles on my Chuck Taylors as we hike along the sandy trail.

"There it is." Catching his breath, Pookie points a little left of the path. "There it is."

"Well that most certainly is a lovely rock," condescendingly I agree. "But I'm really getting hungry."

"Boy shut up," he laughs. "Go climb your ass on top of that rock."

Pookie knew very well that there was no need to instruct me to climb a rock. Show me a rock, or a tree for that matter, and climbing is inevitable. Standing before me, this boulder beckons to be scaled. I reach down extending Pookie my hand and slowly turn around. That's when I see it and immediately I know why, of all the wonderful places in Austin, TX, this is his favorite spot. Perched in a tree overlooking Lake Travis, I remain silent. Stretched on the adjacent boulder, Mike and Pookie gaze down the scenic cliff.

"What do I have to complain about?" I ask myself.

Sometime a new perspective is all we need to appreciate our own beautiful disaster. Leaning back, I run my hands over the tree's scaly bark. It was like the vinyl that cracked along the seats of Pookie's old car. Nothing, however, that a plastic slip cover couldn't fix. I smile for a moment, thinking about the furniture at his childhood home. Pookie's mom slip covered everything. The couch, the chairs, even the lamp shades. "They stay looking new that way," she'd say.

I look over and I see Pookie. It's as if he's dreaming with his eyes wide open.

"Look at this place," he says. "Isn't God great?"

"He certainly is." I agree. Thinking of the many reasons I have to be grateful, I repeat. 'He certainly is. Sometime we just need reminding."

Pookie's outlook on life gives me all the reminding that I need. "What do I have to complain about?" Closing my eyes, I reflect upon my many blessings to a day when it was abundantly clear.

It was a day that started rather crappy. A day that started with me sitting upon the cold travertine tile surrounding the toilet flange chiseling away. Once again, Brett broke the commode. Yet another reason I remind myself that he's eternally twelve. Pulsating through the sewer pipes, Brett's karaoke filled the room. "Living on a Prayer," my ass. The smell of poop was nauseating.

"Can life get any worse than this?" I thought to myself.

Just then, a fragment of PVC pipe popped up and struck me in the eye. Holding my eyelid shut, I staggered to our medicine cabinet. There was an eye wash kit somewhere in the house and we finally had a need for it. Flipping through random first aid products proved to be pointless. A foreign object was lodged in my eye and the case of Pepto-Bismol we bought at Sam's Club would do me no good.

"Hey what's up?" Tilting my head back, I answered my phone.

The worry in my friend's voice made my eyes open wide.

"It's Jonathan." Concerned about her son, my friend continued. "I just don't know what to do."

"What's wrong Pamela?"

"He was out all night. He's been spending the night at random girls' houses and I think he's smoking marijuana."

"Wow!" In disbelief, I exclaimed. "That doesn't sound like him."

"If you only knew…"

A stinging sensation hit me as tears ran down my cheek. "Do you mind if I place the phone down for a moment?" Apologetically, I asked. "I have something in my eye."

"No, go right ahead."

Reaching across the kitchen counter, I grabbed the spray hose adjacent to the sink. Leaning back I squeezed its stainless steel handle. With my head emerged in our kitchen sink, I wished. I wished that my son was out getting laid and smoking pot. Young adults do stupid things. Oh how I wished that Cade was doing such stupid things.

"Sorry about that Pamela." Drying my face with my shirt, I continued. "I'll have a talk with Jonathan."

"Thank you so much. He really admires you."

"No problem. I love that kid." Noticing the water that splashed everywhere, I laughed. "You should see the mess that I made."

I tried my best to keep a straight face as I comforted my friend. While talking her through her predicament, I placed my phone on speaker. There was a big clean up job ahead of me and it required both hands to be free.

"What's that awful noise?" Pamela asked.

"What noise?" Gathering a mop, I rummaged through our laundry room.

"That shrieking sound. Where are you?"

"I'm in the laundry room."

"Oh… OK," she recalled. "I remember you saying that your washing machine was making a lot of noise…but, I thought that you bought a new one."

"Pamela." As I walked past Brett's room I informed her. "That's no washing machine. That dreadful noise," in laughter I continued, "is Brett singing Bon Jovi's greatest hits."

The hard rocking tunes were suddenly overshadowed by the sound of shattered glass.

"Cade!" I yelled as I ran towards the living room.

Fearful of what I'd find, I took a deep breath. There, on the corner of the couch, sat my son. The picture window behind him had been annihilated. There were tears in his eyes as he tightly clenched his fists.

"Need medicine, Daddy."

Later that day, while visiting a friend in the hospital, I received a text message from Pamela.

Pamela: "Is everything all right?…"

> *Me:* "Everything is fine. Cade had a migraine and busted the window. He's feeling much better now…"

Pamela: "Looks like you're dealing with much bigger issues than I am. WTF do I have to complain about?…"

Smiling, I placed my phone back down. My friend Adam was lying in bed rubbing his chest.

"Ain't this some shit?" Pointing to the implant just below his shoulder, Adam explained how his chemotherapy was administered.

Fascinated by medical science, I listened as he continued. "This round lump right here is called a port. There's a tube that connects the port to my vein. When it's time for my chemo, they just inject a needle into the port."

Adam spoke of his chemotherapy and rare cancer the same way that I would speak about lunch or a pair of tennis shoes; like it's no big deal. There's one thing, however, that I knew to be bothering him. Adam's a very active guy and fitness is an integral part of who he is. With wires still connected to the adjacent infusion pole, he nudged his bed to the side. Dropping onto the floor, Adam sneaked in a few push-ups.

Moments later, Adam's parents walked into the room and their faces immediately lit up. Not because their son was on the hospital floor doing push-ups, mind you. But because he had company. This would be my first time meeting Adam's parents. "What an amazing family," I thought as we spent the next several hours laughing and sharing stories in the hospital lobby.

I didn't make it home until 1:00 a.m. that morning. To my surprise, Julee was still sitting up in bed reading a book.

"The window looks worse than I thought," she sighed. "How's Adam?"

Inspired by Adam's courage and positive outlook, I told Julee all about my visit. I told her about the many fascinating things I learned about Adam. I had no idea that Adam was such an incredible artist and musician. I told her about the many fascinating things I learned about Adam's parents. What can I say? They're just downright cool. Realizing what Adam's parents are going through, I gave thanks. I gave thanks for my son's good health. Raising a child with autism can be grueling at times.

However, I am thankful that my son is not battling a life-threatening illness.

"What the fuck do we have to complain about?" I asked as I kissed Julee good night.

The next evening I sent Adam a message.

> *Me:* "Thanks for the inspiration. I went out there to cheer you up and in return you cheered me up. You are the shit my friend."
>
> *Adam:* "Thanks but I ain't nothing special. The cancer patient across the hall from me is blind and has autism. WTF do I have to complain about?"

Opening my eyes, I drift back to reality with a newfound gratefulness. If you've never spent some time reflecting in a tree next to a boulder overlooking a cliff on a lake, I suggest that you give it a try. I promise you won't regret it.

"I'm still hungry," I announce from a high reaching branch.

Tossing a pine cone atop Mike's head, I manage to grab their attention. The three of us drive a few more miles, about two or three songs further I'd say. And that's when we arrive at the Oasis, a Tex-Mex haven promising one of the most remarkable sunsets ever witnessed. They say that everything is bigger in the lone star state and they weren't kidding. The Oasis seats over 2,500 people among multiple levels hugging a rugged cliff along Lake Travis. It's the ideal hot spot for those opposed to climbing up a tree. And what do we have for lunch? Burritos of course.

Lifting our margarita glasses in cheer, we salute…"To friendship."

We make an important pact that day. In tequila, not in blood, we promise to enjoy the simple things in life; to always make time for friends and family; and to never, regardless of life's many obstacles, never give up on our dreams. It's an easy thing to do – to give up on a dream. Slowly, the years pass feeling as if they've been wasted searching for that special something -- that gold medal that could have been ours if only we tried hard enough. Heartache and struggle knock us back a few times, and slowly we change. We convince ourselves that dreams are not important and that we just don't desire them any longer. We strive for the more practical things, like a steady job with a 401K. We want the things that we know we can count on like a reliable sedan with low mileage and an extended warranty. That's what we've become and it's really quite sad. In Austin those smoldering flames were reignited like hot charcoal doused in lighter fluid on a Texas barbeque pit. Pookie always dreamed of being a big Hollywood star. Mike can play a guitar like nobody's business. And as for me, well I've long desired to put this crazy life into writing in hopes of helping others.

"Y'all need to check out Sixth Street tonight," Pookie suggests.

"What do you mean y'all? Aren't you joining us?" I ask.

"Hell no," he replies. "You done wore me out. I had a great time though. I just need to get some rest for tomorrow."

"What do you have planned for us tomorrow?"

"What do I have planned?" He repeats. "I plan to live. The doctor said there's no more cancer in my colon so I just plan to live."

"Dude!" I shout, my voice cracking like a prepubescent kid. "That's great news. You didn't tell me that."

"Well the fight's not over," he explains. "I still have cancer. It's just not in my colon anymore."

Heading back to Pookie's house the volume on the radio creeps progressively louder. Each new breath is a reason to live and each new song is a reason to sing. While stopped in the middle lane of a busy intersection I notice a homeless man at the adjacent corner. He's carrying a sign that reads, "Wife ran off with ninja boyfriend. Need money for karate lessons."

Appreciating life, I find myself struck with the urge to help. I glance up at the red light and then back again at the man with the sign.

"Boy, what are you doing?" Pookie asks. "There's a lot of homeless people in these streets. The sad thing is that if you give him money, he's just going to go buy booze with it."

"Yeah," I shout as I jump out of the vehicle. "But now he can buy the good stuff."

The light turns green and immediately people lay on their horns creating a shitload of noise. Unaffected by their loud commotion, the honking has an odd melodic appeal to me. I adjust my seatbelt and crank the radio a few beats higher. Pookie and Mike sing along with Jason Mraz and I laugh. It's happy hour and I just gave this guy enough money to buy a round for the entire bar. You see, God places people in our lives when we need them most. That man needed a drink and I needed a laugh. It's a beautiful sunny day so I roll the windows down. Extending my hand over the side view mirror, I let the wind carry me away. "I'm Yours" is echoing from the car's speakers. Loud and uncontrollably I join in. Admittedly, my singing is awful but suddenly I really don't care who hears me. You see, each day that we wake up is a gift. That in itself is a reason to sing. And from what I've learned through that mysterious woman on St. Charles Avenue ten years ago, if there's a reason to sing, there's certainly a reason to dance. Listen to the music that God's playing all around us. Each passing note is one beat closer to the end. Our lives are short. Find your reason to dance before the song is over.

Chapter 15

Canned Peaches

We had just finished hauling our waste to the county recycling center. It's one of the little things that we do to save money. Rather than pay a monthly fee for garbage pickup service, I take it there myself.

Here's how it works:

- Garbage cards cost $4 a piece.
- Each card has 4 punches and allows 1-10 bags of garbage
- Each bag of recyclables earns a $2 credit

The goal is to bring enough recyclables to offset the amount of waste. Good recycling habits = free garbage disposal. Placing my unused garbage card back into my wallet, I lean towards Cade.

"So Cade," I ask. "What would you like to do next?"

"Daddy…" pausing he looks back at me. "Go to Starbucks."

Although autism has limited Cade's vocabulary, he's still a rather chatty guy. He stands at the Starbucks counter ready to order his favorite fall treat. Pointing to the barista, Cade shakes his finger while looking over the menu board.

"Hey." Cade says with a smile. "What's your name?"

"Dylan," replies the young man. Eyes level with Cade, his frame is lean. About 100 pounds lighter I'd say. "What's your name?"

"Cade." He smiles in his usual awkward manner. Squinting his eyes, his grin stretches across his face. With a smile from ear to ear, his eyes close and then open wide again. "Dylan…" He pauses before he queries. "Are you happy?"

"Yes Cade," he replies. "I'm very happy."

"Dylan…" Again Cade pauses. "Do you have a dog?"

"I do have a dog."

"What's your dog's name?"

"His name is Ace."

"Ace is a boy?" Cade says with a question.

"Ace is a boy." Dylan confirms.

"Dylan…"

Cade proceeds through his usual series of questioning. And if we never see Dylan again, Cade will always remember every detail of this young man. He'll remember his name. He'll remember his dog's name. He'll remember his birthday. And he'll even remember his kitchen appliances.

Before long, caffeine seeking patrons enter the door. With both of my hands on the back of Cade's head, I shift his attention back to the menu board.

"What would you like?" I ask.

"Pumpkin Spice Latte." He loudly cheers. Ordering done, he steps aside. "…and a pumpkin scone."

We sit on the soft leather chairs, Cade and I. Anxiously, Cade awaits his name to be called.

"Tall Non-Fat Latte for Brenda."

A well-manicured hand reaches for the cup. As she lifts the warm beverage, she slips it into an insulated sleeve.

"Brenda…" Cade gets her attention. "Are you happy?"

"I'm happy now." With her beverage in hand, she says goodbye.

"Grande Caramel Macchiato for John."

"John…" Cade approaches. "Are you happy?"

Without fail, the first thing Cade asks when meeting someone is, "Are you happy?"

Oddly enough, Julee and I still aren't allowed to say "happy." We always refer to it as the "H" word. The most common word in Cade's vocabulary becomes shady when we use it. Therefore, we treat the "H" word like we treat those questionable friends that are always trying to sell their multi-level marketing crap. We avoid it by all means necessary.

You see, it all started several years ago when Cade first started experiencing migraines. With limited words, he couldn't formulate, "It feels like my skull exploded and a leprechaun is stabbing me in the fucking eye with an ice pick." Instead, he'd scream while referring to himself in the third person. "You're not HAP-PY! You're not HAP-PY!" Since then, Julee and I are forbidden from using the "H" word. It's become a trigger of sorts for Cade.

So what does the "H" word trigger these days? Let's go back to those soft leather chairs at the local Starbucks. They're quite comfortable. It's a beautiful Saturday afternoon. I had just checked the monthly trip to the recycling center off my to-do list and I'm feeling spectacularly cleansed. For some reason, I get this feeling every time that I leave the dump. It's the same way that I feel the morning after drinking a cup of Smooth Move tea. Cade greets everyone passing by and I tap my feet joyfully to the music. Leaning back, Cade pulls his phone from the side pocket of his cargo pants.

"That's so gross Cade!" I shriek.

"Dad..." Licking the froth above his lip, he laughs. "You watching Dr. Pimple Popper."

And so Cade indulges in pumpkin scones, pimples, blackheads and giant boils. With both hands on the back of my own head, I shift my attention away. To get my mind off the massive puss filled extraction I just witnessed, I focus on the music. I must say, I do love Pharrell Williams. Shortly into the chorus, I begin singing along and that's when the "H" word comes out. "How stupid!" I think to myself. After all, the name of the damn song is "Happy." Immediately, I shut my mouth. My eyes drift towards Cade and I wait for his outburst. Questioningly, he looks back at me. For some reason, however, he remains captivated with Dr. Pimple Popper. I actually got away with saying the "H" word; or so I thought. Cade takes another bite of his scone and I scroll through social media.

Facebook, the place where people treat each other like the trash that I take to the dump. The place where people post ten or so hate filled rants followed by "Jesus is my savior. Type 'Amen' if you agree." It doesn't take a genius to know that this type of thinking only applies to household waste. And while one bag of recyclables may offset five or more bags of garbage, one pleasant post does not do the same. Hate is hate. There's no number of puppies, kittens, grandchildren or spiritual memes that can offset hate. Shaking my head, I turn off social media and turn on Dr. Pimple Popper. I'll take a nasty cyst over a nasty human any day.

Cade takes a final bite of his scone. Still sitting in his chair, he abruptly stomps his feet. The front of his shirt is pulled over to the back of his head. His face stretches through the fabric like a Pin Art toy you'd see on an executive's desk. With his belly fully exposed he begins to scream. "HAP-PY! ... HAP-PY! ... HAP-PY! ...HAP-PY!

So the next time that you see a grown man watching Dr. Pimple Popper while sitting next to an individual screaming the "H" word with his shirt pulled over his head, relax. It's pumpkin season.

We head back home, Cade and I with autumn treats to share. As we approach the house, I notice Brett running along the driveway. He turns the corner to the front sidewalk and our newly planted mums bite the dust. We go inside and place the Starbucks bag onto the countertop. My back hurts from lifting the large branches that we hauled to the dump earlier this morning.

"Hey Tote!" I yell for Brett. "I have a pumpkin muffin for you."

He doesn't answer.

"Hey Tote!" Again I call.

"Oooohhh..." He comes strolling through the kitchen in his Jack Skellington boxer shorts and high top tennis shoes.

"Oh I love pumpkin muffins." He smiles and opens the bag. "Oh look, a cake pop. I love cake pops even more. I'll take that instead."

"What happened to the flowers Julee just planted in the front?" I ask.

"Oh, I didn't do that."

"Do what?"

"Run over those flowers. Someone else must have done that."

"I guess you're right Brett." I tell him. "It must have been someone else then."

Content with his cake pop, Brett turns to go back into his room.

"Hey Twont," he turns back towards me. "Why didn't you get me a coffee?"

"I didn't think about it Brett. I just thought you might like a pastry."

"Well, it's Okay," he tells me. "I'm not mad."

I take a muffin to Julee and laugh. She's sitting in the living room reading a book.

"What ae you reading?" I ask.

"*Does the Noise in my Head Bother You?*" She abruptly replies.

"Somebody's a little grumpy today. Maybe I should have gotten you a grumpkin muffin instead."

Turning the book cover toward me she rolls her eyes and grins. "*Does the Noise in my Head Bother You?* It's a memoir written by Steven Tyler." Biting into her 'grumpkin' muffin, she gives me a condescending look. "Well at least you're pretty."

In agreeance I nod my head. She just smiles and goes on about what an interesting man Steven Tyler is. Flipping the pages of her book, she tells me about the Aerosmith front man's epic life on the road and the relationship that he has with his children. I smile as Julee gives me an abridged version of the legendary rock star.

"Shall we dance?" I ask.

I Google Aerosmith ballads and in small circles we sway to "Dream On." I've always been more of a swayer than a dancer. There's less coordination required.

"Remember us?" She asks.

Her head leans softly onto my chest. My body moves slowly, trying to keep in pace with the music. There's an awkwardness to my dance moves, but in this point in time I really don't care. It's within these carefree moments that you fall in love and it's within these carefree moments that you stay in love. Just like life, our dance is far from perfect. It is, however, familiar. And there's something rather spectacular in familiarity

The song comes to an end and we continue swaying. "Love in an Elevator" isn't exactly my idea of a ballad and before long I let go. Jumping onto the coffee table, I take center stage. Just like brother-in-law Brett, I too am a rock star.

"Hey scuba squat!" I yell.

Brett doesn't reply so I dash quickly across the house and bust open his bedroom door. Turning his head sharply, he keeps his train of thought. His "Crazy Train" that is. In tune with his inner Osbourne, Brett continues belting the classic metal lyrics. I grab Brett's Play Station guitar and just like that, an Ozzy / Aerosmith mashup is born. For the next two hours I'm a member of Brett's awesome rock band. I rotate among the various Play Station instruments while Brett remains steady on vocals. Who can argue with a voice like that?

"Well it was nice rocking out with you," Brett tells me. "But *Law & Order* is about to come on."

Taking his cue, I place my drum sticks down and bid farewell.

"Yeah..." Holding my head down like a heartbroken puppy I continue, "It was nice rocking out with you too."

I exit Brett's room and Julee stands before me. She has the most beautiful smile and those eyes, those caramel colored eyes.

"You know," she tells me. "It really means a lot to him."

"Who?" I ask. "That tote?"

"Yeah…" Her smile extends. "That tote."

I look into her eyes and instantly I'm reminded of the night that we first met.

It was Club Seventeen, a teenage nightclub in St. Bernard Parish, where we met. She wore one lace glove and a black bustier that covered her form fitting t-shirt. The year was 1986. Chalmette was a small town in a post-Madonna *Like a Virgin* era.

Before the evening that the slim guy in baggy pants and Duran Duran hair asked her to dance, it was just Julee and her group of girlfriends. Julee was a huge Cyndi Lauper fan. And although *Girls Just Want to Have Fun* she would fuck up anyone that messed with her little brother.

"Kelly." I extended my fingerless gloved hand. Like opposing magnetic poles, our hands connected.

"Julee," she continued, "with two e's." Lightly, she pulled back. Unexplainably, however, our hands remain locked.

That's when I first noticed her eyes. Although the air was brisk on that crowded balcony, Julee's eyes were warm and inviting -- the color of my favorite McDonald's sundae topping. Again, she lightly pulled her hand back.

"I think our gloves are stuck." She giggled.

"What?" Bending my wrist back, I continued, "I'm sorry."

There I stood in my baggy pants as she gently peeled her lace from the Velcro strap of my leather glove.

"There... Now you're free," she said.

"Thanks," I replied.

But I was far from free. With my heart held captive, I followed Julee to the dance floor. I truly wasn't much for dancing. I never understood why anyone would purposely convulse in public. Who'd want to create such a spectacle anyway? The strange thing is that I was always a class clown. And although I would willingly make an absolute ass of myself for a laugh; dancing, for some reason, frightened the crap out of me.

"I love this song," she shouted.

"Who doesn't?" I thought to myself. After all, it is Prince.

Bouncing to the upbeat tempo of the hit song "Kiss," Julee twirled and ran her fingers across my shoulder. Taking her signal, my right foot began to move. To awaken my left foot, she slid her right foot forward. A few gentle taps and my entire body was set into motion. Soon my inhibitions vanished and my vocals spanned an octave range only His Royal Badness could achieve. At least that's what I'd like to think. When all is said and done, who would attempt to sing a Prince song any other way?

Despite my dreadful singing and dancing, Julee hung around for more. Stepping off the dance floor, we ordered a couple drinks. A non-alcoholic strawberry daiquiri for her and a Coca Cola for me; this was the start of our new life. Julee was very animated when she spoke. She reminded me, of all things, Minnie Mouse. Her face lit up with pure enchantment as she told me about her hobbies, about the music that she loved and about her favorite books and movies. And that's when she told me about her dream job. She hoped to one day be able to drive the tram at Walt Disney World's Magic Kingdom.

Holding our opaque plastic cups we sat in a corner booth. It was a dimly lit hot spot with a little less noise. Spilled Shirley Temples and bubble gum coated the tables and seats. Sticky was as much of the atmosphere as synthesized pop music. With a napkin from the tabletop dispenser, I wiped the best that I could. Licking my thumb, I buffed away at the syrupy surface.

"That's really sweet," she said with a generous smile.

"Yeah," I concurred. "And sticky too."

"That's not what I meant." In laughter she went on. "Now tell me about you."

And so I let her know all of my crazy dreams. Dreams, which for once did not seem out of reach. Julee made me feel, at that moment, that anything was possible. Therefore, she deserved to know the truth.

"I'm not the best dancer." Lowering my head in shame, I confessed.

"You're kidding me, right?"

"No," I answered. "Unfortunately, it's true."

"Well I would have never known."

And anything was possible. Anything other than me learning to dance, that is. The two of us sat next to each other in our cozy corner booth. On the one clean spot among the grimy tabletop stood our two Dixie cups and sticky napkin shreds. For someone with no dance skills, I knew that I had to be smooth.

"You want to see me drink this Coke with no hands?"

"No." She wrinkled her nose at me and laughed.

"Sure you do."

With my hands held behind my back I lowered my head. As my teeth firmly gripped the curled edges of the plastic rim, I tilted my head back and down went the beverage -- not a drop wasted.

"Well that's impressive," she reluctantly uttered.

Silently, and without any slurping she sipped through her plastic straw. She had a way, even then, of subtly teaching me proper etiquette.

"Do you like to read?" she asked me with a smile in her eyes.

"Sure," I nodded. "Reading… I love reading."

"What have you read lately?"

"Well, honestly I'm more of a *CliffsNotes* kind of guy."

"So you don't read?" again she asked.

"Of course I read," I professed. "I read just enough to pass the test. Hence, my love for *CliffsNotes*."

I may not have been able to win her over with intellectual book discussions, but I did make her laugh. And laughter, like Walt Disney himself, creates magic of its very own. She leaned in closer resting her chin upon her lace glove. Without hesitation, I followed her lead and softly our lips touched. The kiss itself may have been small. But the side effects were huge. And although I had never been high, I imagined that this was what it felt like. Suddenly my head filled with fireworks and in a loopy daze I walked her back to the dance floor.

New Edition's "Is This the End" signaled that the evening was almost over. On any given weekend night, this was the last track played at Club Seventeen. The two of us danced until the very last note and then we went our separate ways. As Julee walked back to her car, I walked over to Pookie's car. Leaning against the trunk of his baby blue Pinto I glanced back towards Julee. The gleam in her caramel eyes gave me all the strength that I needed. Turning myself around, I briskly pushed that piece of shit car down the street.

"All right Pookie," I yelled. "You can pop the clutch now!"

And from that moment on, I knew that she was the one that I wanted to grow old with. Well, at least I'd grow old and she'd stay the same age. "The hardest part in lying about your age," she'd say, "is remembering how old you really are."

My phone rings and I run to pick it up.

"It's Pookie," I announce to Julee before saying hello.

"Hey man! I was just thinking about you and the nights that we'd hangout at Club Seventeen. How are you?"

"I'm good," Pookie replies in an unconvincing manner.

It's sort of like one of those automatic out of office email messages. We all do it. When someone asks us how we're doing, there's a 90% chance that they're going to hear "fine." But it's different among friends and something just doesn't sound right.

"You sure?"

"Yes," he assures me. "I'm just tired."

"Your treatments going all right?" I ask.

"I'm done with my chemo."

"Well that's good..." I pause for a moment. "Right?"

"Yeah," sluggishly he continues. "It's good for now. I just wish I could make it to Tyler's football game. His team is playing in the Georgia Dome next week and the doctor said I shouldn't be traveling. He said I have a high risk of infection."

"Sorry brother." Searching for the right words to say, again I pause. "Cancer sucks!"

"Yes it does." He agrees.

"Yeah," Like Mickey Goldmill pumping up Rocky Balboa in the corner ring, I cheer him on. "Fuck cancer!"

Pookie doesn't say anything for a few moments. But when he does, I can hear his smile.

"Besides," I reassure him, "Atlanta is not that far of a drive for me. I'll be there for Tyler. And he knows that you'd be there too if you could."

"Thanks brother. It really means a lot to me."

A week later I wake up early for our trip to Atlanta. While whipping up a special treat, I transform myself into Donkey from the movie *Shrek*.

"Here you go Cade...parfait"

Digging his spoon into the mountain of goodness, Cade replies as the big green ogre. I love that Cade knows all of the lines to so many movies. Laughing to myself, I get to work. With my hands in the sink and my head in the clouds, I scrub away. It's time to catch up on the dishes. Watching through the opening I observe him. Cade's wearing his favorite *Teenage Mutant Ninja Turtles* t-shirt. His eyes reflect the morning sun filtering through our picture window.

"Mmmm…"

Cade scoops through the top layer. But then again, who doesn't love whipped cream? Adoringly, I watch my son smile; a gift that I cherish so much. While scribbling on a sheet of construction paper, he licks the corner of his mouth.

"Wow Cade! Is that the Incredible Hulk?"

"Yeah…"

Cade admires his artwork as his superhero progresses. Laying down his crayon, he moves on to the next layer. As his spoon digs deeper, it's suddenly the best of both worlds. Bits of cake and ice cream dance along Cade's palate. Several crayon strokes later and his masterpiece comes to life.

"Great job Cade." I applaud. "That's one bad ass Hulk drawing."

"Yes." He so proudly agrees. "I know."

Rewarding himself, Cade dives into the depths of his dessert glass. As I watch him I'm not prepared for what's coming next. He has never been fond of canned peaches, my buddy. And quickly his taste buds sour.

"Yuk!" Cade exclaims as he spits across the table.

"Yuk!" Also replies the Hulk pounding the preserved fruit into submission. "Hulk smash!" He roars.

In all honesty, I had forgotten about Cade's disdain towards canned peaches. You see, Cade doesn't exemplify hate. It's part of the beauty of his innocence. Although he's becoming a young man, autism has kept him very much a child. And quite simply, children don't know hate. Children learn hate. They learn it by the actions of those they admire. They learn it from us. This trip to Atlanta would remind me of just that.

Tyler's mom and step dad are hosting a party to honor their amazing children. Unfortunately, I don't get to see Tyler and Summer as often as I wish. Hurricane Katrina has placed miles between so many friends and family. However, when we do get together, we just pick up where we left off.

Together, we sit at the patio table indulging in crawfish and comradery. Proud of Tyler's outstanding achievements, I glance towards him. With mutual respect, together we nod our heads. The DJ spins, the crowd mingles and the little ones ravage the bounce house. The shaded back yard was providing for an enjoyable day in the otherwise hot Georgia sun.

Before long, a couple of uninvited guests arrive. Two young Caucasian boys were playing in the woods behind the house. Their adolescent adventures led them to the celebration that was taking place. Curiously, they climb across the fence. "Brave move," I think as they intermix among the crowd. Within moments Tyler's step father approaches the two inquisitive youths. Their eyes roll upwards acknowledging the man's towering presence. Tyler's step father is from the south and he isn't about to have uninvited guests wandering about his home. Not without a plate of food and a large chunk of cake, that is. The two adventurers spend the remainder of the afternoon meeting new people, laughing and having a bayou style good time. As they head back across the fence, Tyler's step father stops them once more. You see Tyler's step father is from the south and he isn't about to have uninvited guests leave his home empty handed. They part ways with new friends, new stories and a bag of hot boiled crawfish.

So here's to the beauty of a child's innocence. My son has never known a difference between him and Tyler. To Cade, skin pigmentation is of no significance. To Cade, we're all the same.

My son has no preconceived judgment of race, color, religion, national origin, sex, sexuality nor disability. To Cade, it's all insignificant. To Cade, we're all the same. And although Cade and Tyler are close in age, Uncle Pookie and I are much older. To Cade, age is of no significance. To Cade, we're all the same. We're all just teenagers in the eyes of my son.

What would you do differently if you had the chance to be a teenager again? Everyday Cade makes me strive to be a better person. His open heart acceptance is absolutely inspiring. A little kindness really does go a long way. After all, we're all worthy of so much more than canned peaches.

Chapter 16

Our Heavenly Home

There's a couple seats near the front of the theater, aisle seats nonetheless. The perfect spot for a trip to the movies with Cade. Outings with autism are always best when carefully planned. Our seating of choice remains the location that provides the easiest escape in the event of a meltdown. We take our seats, my buddy and I. Leaning over a big ass tub of popcorn I whisper, "Who's gonna win?"

"Batman," he replies.

The caped crusader is by far Cade's favorite. *The Dark Knight Rises* had just made its way to the discount cinema. And although this is the second time watching the film for both of us, it's our first time seeing it together. Cade first saw the film in July during his summertime with Nana.

Physically, Cade appears to be an adult -- a rather large adult rivaling the size of many among the DC Universe. However, within his towering facade lies a small child. Cade's the tortoise and the hare wrapped into one fantastically complicated fable. Hopeful that slow and steady wins the race; I long for the day that Cade progresses emotionally past a four-year-old. Until then, I remain the parent of an individual old enough to know better, but young enough to not care. Doing as a four-year-old does Cade loudly announces, "Restroom, Daddy."

"But we just went to the restroom buddy." I respond. "Why didn't you go then?"

"Restroom, Daddy," he repeats.

Doing as the parent of a four-year-old does, I escort him to the restroom. Exiting the theater I place my 3D glasses above my head and Cade does the same. It's the usual restroom visit: #1 or #2 followed by hand washing and waving side to side in front of a dryer sensor that doesn't work. Wiping my hands on my pants I glance in the mirror. My 3D glasses have disheveled my coif. With my hands above my head praying mantis style, I work my hair back to the way that I like it. Messy but not too messy; it's my idea of controlling the uncontrollable. Cade stands next to me with perfectly-styled light chestnut locks. He has been blessed with a thick head of hair that just stays put. Observing me, he becomes a young praying mantis and he does the same. Messy but not too messy; the two of us head back to our seats.

    My hands are always cold. Julee says it's like sleeping with a vampire. Cade, on the other hand, is very warm natured. He takes after his mother in that manner. I place my hands beneath my thighs to keep them warm and I lean my head back. Cade's eyes remain locked straight ahead as his idol emerges on the screen. Noticing me through his peripheral vision, Cade places his hands beneath his thighs and he leans his head back. Together, the two of us enjoy the show.

    It's a weekday evening so the theater's not so crowded. Cade stays mesmerized as comic book legends battle on the big screen. Immersed in superhero bliss, he remains focused.

    "Beat his ass, Batman!" Cade shouts to the screen.

    "Shhh..." I lean over once more. "Let's use our inside voice."

    "Beat... his... ass," he slowly and softly repeats.

    Excited that Cade actually used volume control, I gave him kudos. "Great job with that inside voice, Doo-Doo."

    I still call Cade Doo-Doo from time to time. I don't know why. I just do.

    "Bump it bro!" I tell him.

We exchange a fist bump and get back to the movie. I cross my arms in front of me and Cade does the same. They say that mirroring is a subconscious behavior. They say that we imitate the gestures, both verbal and nonverbal, of those that surround us. This is especially true of our closest friends and family. Cade, on the other hand mimics my every move in a very conscious and purposeful manner. Even in a room full of super heroes, he's watching my every move. It's clear to me that if I want Cade to be a better person, then I must be a better person as well. My father used to always tell me, "Don't do as I do. Do as I say." And while I didn't do as he did, it was because I was smart enough to know better.

We live in a world where we think we can change people through insults. For some reason we believe that calling individuals childish names will make them somehow see things our way. This is the same dumb ass mentality of drivers with road rage. On the highway as well as in life, sometime they're the assholes and sometime we're the assholes. If we expect others to take it easy when we unintentionally cut them off, then we must do the same. For it's in our most frustrating and challenging moments that it's most important to lead by example. Show them a better way. There's no telling who's watching. As far as the childish name calling, I say leave the jokes for the comedians. In a world full of Jokers, be something bigger. Be the Batman!

We get back home and Mr. Yang is waiting at the gate.

"Feed me," he instructs telepathically.

"Yang," I tell him. "You sure don't look like you've missed any meals. Do you expect me to believe that I'm the only neighbor you're giving those sad eyes to?"

"Meow," replies Yang stroking along the picket gate.

Don't Squeeze the Spaceman's Taco

Cade tosses Yang some leftover popcorn. Oddly enough, the cat enjoys it. We go inside the house and I grab a can of tuna. Let's just say that I'm a pushover for all things furry.

"Here you go Yang." I place a paper plate on the back steps. "The tuna was on sale, buy one get one free. I sure hope you like Bumble Bee."

In a display of gratitude, the cat bows his head and then slams his face into the mound before him.

The next morning Mr. Yang returns the favor. Julee screams and slams the door. She catches her breath and then quiets down.

"There's a dead mouse on the back step."

I smile discreetly and then get up. Bugs and dead rodents have long been my job.

"I'll go get it."

I walk back into the kitchen following Operation Dead Mouse Disposal. Julee is in the bedroom getting ready for work.

"Thanks for taking care of that," she yells through the closed door.

"You're welcome," I reply. "I'm making your breakfast."

"You're so sweet...I sure hope you washed your hands."

"Of course," condescendingly I answer while delivering her a cup of coffee. "Here you go. Just the way you like it. Half and half with a teaspoon of sugar."

"Thank you Biscuit. You're too good to me."

"Yeah," I agree. "This is true."

"It's really been great having you at home." She looks at me lovingly and grins. "I think I'm getting spoiled."

I have to agree with her. It has been great staying at home. It's allowed me to give Cade the attention that he so desperately needed. Heck, my cooking has even improved. When it comes to cooking, I've learned that as long as I stick to the recipe and do as instructed, the food isn't half bad. Who knew? My cooking, however, is still reserved for those weekday quick meals. Weekends and holidays are when Julee runs the kitchen. And with the Thanksgiving holiday approaching, that's one of my many reasons to be thankful.

My phone rings so I go to the bedroom where it's charging and pick it up.

"I have bad news." Remembering the last time that Pookie uttered those four words, I cringe.

"What's going on?" I ask while holding my breath.

"I'm not able to make it out there to see y'all this Thanksgiving."

Relieved, I exhale. "That's not a problem," I tell him. "We'll just do Thanksgiving in Texas… and I promise, no burritos."

"I don't think I'll be home either."

I close my eyes and search my head for positive thoughts. My hand trembles as I hold the phone tightly against my ear.

"You didn't end up on the wrong side of one of those prison cells that you guard, did you?"

"Boy you need to shut up?" Pookie laughs then quiets down and coughs. "I almost wish that I did."

"Well that's good news," I continue. "And all this time you told me that you had bad news."

We go on for a bit keeping everything light hearted. And then the heaviness hits.

"I'm in hospice care."

Suddenly I lose my breath. My heart is pounding as I struggle to comprehend what I'm hearing. "How could this be?" I ask myself. "Pookie was making such big strides at defeating his cancer." With tears rolling down my cheeks, I do my best to disguise the sadness that consumes me.

"Hospice care is a wonderful thing." I assure him. My fist clenches my St. Jude medal as I battle to assure myself. 'You're in good hands."

"I know," he agrees. "They've been great to me here. I understand what your cousin Michael meant when he said that hospice can be beautiful."

"That was just last Thanksgiving." Closing my eyes, the past year flashes before me.

"I know." With a light chuckle he continues, "It's been one hell of a year."

"It really has." Still clenching my medal I repeat, "It really has."

Pookie's light chuckle transforms into roaring laughter and all of a sudden the heaviness is lifted. Laughter is contagious and before long I'm cracking up.

"What kind of drugs do they have you on over there?" I ask with a hint of sarcasm.

"Morphine," he continues to laugh. "But it's not that."

"Well then, what's so funny?"

"Last Thanksgiving," Pookie continues. "You've got me thinking about last Thanksgiving." He clears his throat and then nails one hell of an Aunt Delores impression. "I sure do love that Pookie… You know, he doesn't act B-L-A-C-K."

Shortly after hanging up, the blaring siren from our smoke detector echoes throughout the house. In a mad rush, I scramble to the kitchen. The pan is sizzling and small flames are rising from its center. With a firm grip on the handle, I dunk the pan into the sink.

"What happened?" Julee asks.

"Breakfast," I reply.

"It's all right," noticing the tears in my eyes, she comforts me. "I'll just pick up something on my way to work."

That's when I tell her the news. Dazed and deaf to the piercing alarm, we drop to the ground. Together we sit on the floor of our smoke-filled kitchen and weep. Pookie's been a part of my family since before Julee and I met. They say that blood is thicker than water. I say that they've never seen the waters along the bayou. The friends that you make down Bayou Road are the friends that you keep for life. And a friend for life – well, that's just family.

The next morning I board a plane for Austin, TX; a city that encourage folks to keep it weird. Death, it certainly does keep things weird. It's weird how death reminds us to live. It's weird how facing death requires courage and accepting death requires grace. I arrive at the hospice facility in my budget class economy car. For twenty minutes I sit silently in the shaded lot. "Stay positive…Stay positive…Stay positive…" I shuffle through my iTunes account seeking inspiration from Jason Mraz – a happy moment from my last visit. Five replays of "I'm Yours" and I'm ready to see my best friend. I adjust the brim of my Superman baseball cap and exit the vehicle.

Humming the song that's in my head, I walk the corridor to the nurses' station.

"How may I help you today?" She asks with a smile.

"What's her song?" Quietly, I ask myself. "How many times did she have to press replay before walking in here today?"

"What can we do for you Mr. Kent?" She asks.

"Huh?" Confused, I look her way.

"Clark Kent..." She chuckles and addresses me once more.

"Oh," like a rookie in outfield surprised to actually catch a ball, I awkwardly laugh. "My hat – you're talking about my hat." I stutter a moment and continue, "I'm here to see my friend, Pookie... umm, Dwayne... I mean Marcel... Marcel Weathers. I'm here to see Marcel Weathers."

"We just love Mr. Weathers. He's down the hall to the left -- room number 15."

As I head to Pookie's room near the end of the hallway, a young man dressed in full cowboy gear passes me by. "Howdy," he announces while tipping his hat. There's a miniature pony following just a few steps behind.

Through the open door to my right, I see a teenage girl strumming a ukulele. Singing a carefree song that she wrote to an elderly woman lying in bed, she bobs her head. I continue on towards the end of the hallway. As I approach Pookie's room, I adjust my hat once more and clear my throat. It's a quarter past 11:00 a.m. when I tap on his door.

"Come in," a familiar voice welcomes me.

Taking a deep breath, I step into Pookie's room. My happy song echoes throughout my head. I pump up my internal volume to keep from sobbing at Pookie's frail skeletal appearance. The vibrant, dimple-faced man that I call my brother has literally dwindled to skin and bones. I remind myself to focus on our many good times. The last thing Pookie would want to hear is how much I'm going to miss him. There's a nurse tending to the room. She grabs his soiled linens and leaves.

"Enjoy your visit," she says with a friendly glance. "Mr. Weathers, if you need me just press the nurse button and like magic, I'll appear."

I search for the right things to say and then immediately beat myself up.

"How are you doing?" I ask.

"How's he doing?" Silently and frustratingly, I reply to myself. "He's dying. What kind of question is that?"

"I'm fine." He adjusts his bed to an upright seated position. "It sure is good to see you."

"It's great seeing you too."

"Tell me you rented a nicer car this time."

"Nope," I say. "This one even has manual crank windows." We laugh together a moment and then I continue. "But I got a really good deal."

Pookie reaches through the rail guard along his bed. I grasp his hand and lean in close.

"Thank you for being my friend," he tells me.

His words come out slowly, as if talking has become a strenuous task. There's a plastic bedpan beside him. He turns his head and spits up a bit.

"I am the one that should be thanking you." Admiringly I reply. "But you don't have to throw up just thinking about me."

We continue laughing and then Pookie takes a break. Leaning back, he takes a shallow breath. I observe him lying in bed as he looks wide-eyed towards the ceiling. Little by little his dimples start to emerge.

"Is that a smile?" I ask.

"Yeah," he replies with a rattling whisper.

"What are you thinking about?"

"Life," again he whispers. "I've had a good life."

I grab the lip balm beside his bed and gesture towards him. Pookie nods his head, "yes." Gently, I tap my finger along his dry, chapped lips.

"There," I tell him, "now you can really smile."

And so he does. It's the same smile I remember when he finally passed math class. Still holding his hand, I pull over a chair with my foot. I take off my hat and collapse into the leather cushion.

"Good Lord," he declares. "What happened to you?"

"I did a little remodeling." I reply.

There's Saran wrap around my head to keep my scalp moist. It's only been a few days since my recent hair transplant.

"I moved some hair from the back to the front." I tell him.

"Good," he says. "I didn't want to tell you; but your forehead was getting too damn big."

"Yes it was," I agree and snicker.

"Does it hurt?"

"You know," I reply. "It kind of feels like a hairy tattoo."

Pookie leans back and stares upward towards the ceiling again.

"How often do you talk to your mom?" He asks me.

"Almost every day lately," I tell him.

"That's really nice." Quietly, he gazes to the sky.

I watch over Pookie as he's lying in bed. A few minutes in silence and his face begins to beam. His gauntness can barely constrain those famous dimples of his.

"Read me your mom's poem," he murmurs.

And that's when my tears start falling. Somehow, I remained strong until that moment. Jason Mraz is blasting throughout my brain but I just can't stop crying. Blurry eyed, I scroll through the collection on my phone. My mother's poetry is very dear to me. Although Mom had written many poems throughout the years, I understood Pookie's vague request. For there's one poem that many consider to be Mom's best and I will never forget the day that I discovered it.

I was just seventeen at the time, a senior in high school. Mom had been recently admitted to the hospital for a mild bladder infection.

"The doctor wants to run a few tests," she called to tell me. "But I'll be home soon."

Three days later, I found myself staring at the phone. Mom's bladder infection had progressed into septic shock. Iris and my dad were standing bedside around the clock.

"Yoo-hoo," the front door swung open as Vivian let herself in. "I made you boys some chicken gumbo."

Vivian carried the heavy pot to our kitchen and placed it on the stove.

"Hello Ms. Mary." She greeted my grandmother.

Mémère Mary had been staying with us while Mom was in the hospital.

"Hello Vivian," she replied. "That's very sweet of you."

"Oh it's nothing. I was thinking about y'all over here and I said to myself, 'Let me make them some gumbo.' I've been praying for Helen."

"Oh thank you," replied Mémère. "You think she'll be all right?"

"Do you believe in prayer?" Vivian asked.

"Yes."

"Well, then she's going to be fine. I know that Helen believes in prayer and I know that she believes in miracles too."

A miracle was desperately needed. The next few days were consumed with prayer, uncertainty and creole cooking. The women in my neighborhood shared a common moto: "Feed a cold. Feed a fever. Feed the blues." Vivian's gumbo and Maude's butter beans were like Prozac on our worrisome palates. There's a certain comfort that comes from a home cooked meal.

The next morning Dad came home to take a shower. Apparently Iris told him that he was beginning to stink. Concerned that he'd miss the moment when Mom opened her eyes, he was in and out of the bathroom within minutes. A wave of Vitalis hair tonic and Brut by Faberge trailed behind him.

"Sit down Casie," insisted Maw-Maw Tonia. "You need to eat."

Aunt Gloria had driven my grandmother over knowing that Dad was on the way. Aunt Gloria was a rather cautious driver, but put her on a time crunch and you'd swear that she was running moonshine. The two of them made it with enough time for Maw-Maw Tonia to cook a full breakfast – a foot high stack of golden pancakes, sunny side up eggs, a pot of grits and of course fried shrimp; because my dad loved fried shrimp with his grits.

That afternoon I joined my father back at the hospital. The rain blasted against our windshield. Sudden thunderstorms in St. Bernard Parish were about as common as white rubber boots. Shrimp boots, that's what they called them. For many St. Bernard Parish residents, shrimp boots were the footwear of choice. The polyblend waterproof galoshes were worn to restaurants, grocery stores and even to church. Except of course on Christmas and Easter Sunday. These were the two days out of the year when Jesus noticed your feet. Water beaded along Dad's Vitalis ladened wavy hair as we entered through the glass doors.

"How's Mom?" I asked my sister.

"She's still in a coma." Extending her hand, my sister lifted my chin. "But I know that she can hear me."

"How can you tell?"

"I just know," she replied. "Let's go see her."

The hospital corridor was long and cold. Perhaps it was because I was soaking wet. My feet sloshed in my sneakers as we trekked towards the intensive care unit. My sister opened the door and I walked into Mom's room. Aside from the wires and tubes crossing in every direction, Mom just looked as if she were sound asleep.

"Tell her that you're here," insisted my sister.

"But she's sleeping." I replied.

"Here," tugging at my arm Iris led me to Mom's bedside. "Now hold her hand."

Nervously I placed Mom's hand in mine. It was as if I was afraid to break her. Standing at her side, my cold shivers stopped.

"Go ahead," Iris repeated. "Tell her that you're here."

Clutching Mom's fingertips within my hand, I spoke in a hushed tone.

"Hi Mom."

Uncertain of what to say, I took a deep breath and glanced Iris's way. With a slight nudge of her head, my sister's instructions were clear – keep talking.

"It's me…Kelly…Dad brought me here."

There was a slight movement in her index finger; a twitch maybe. But it was just enough to make my heart flutter.

"Man you should have heard him fussing at the people driving in the rain." With a soft chuckle I leaned in closer. "What a grumpy bastard!"

That's when I knew that it was more than just a twitch. Mom's fingers curled inward as if embracing my hand. There was a bit of a trembling to her movement. In all honesty, it may have been me that was trembling. Gently stroking Mom's hair, I told her about my grumpy father. I told her about the neighbors cooking us meals and checking on us daily. I told her about Mémère Mary staying with us and taking care of our house. Although Mom had tubes running up her nose providing oxygen, she was breathing on her own. At that moment, I knew that she was breathing easier. There's an undeniable peace in knowing that your children are going to be all right.

As soon as I got home that night I prayed. The next morning when I woke up I prayed. Day in and day out over the next week I prayed. I prayed for Mom to return home to us.

But Mom never did. Sobbing, I watched as she took her last breath. I stared at the up and down movement of her chest hoping that it would continue. Hoping that the ventilator she'd recently been placed on was no longer needed. Hoping and praying for a miracle. But my prayers went unanswered. Mom's latest brain scan showed no activity. Faced with the decision to remove Mom's life support, Dad broke down.

Teary-eyed, I helped gather Mom's belongings. Tucked in a drawer beside her bed were possessions that she held dearly. There was a rosary that Maw-Maw Tonia gave her for her 40th birthday; her wedding ring which she had removed when her hands started swelling in the hospital bed; and a thin spiral notebook crinkled around the edges with a ball point pen attached to its cover.

Although the room was now empty, I knew that I wasn't alone. A guiding force told me to be seated. Still angry that Mom wasn't going home and angry that God ignored my prayers, I opened the beat up notebook. I sat there a moment flipping through the wrinkled pages hoping for a sign. But the pages were all blank. All but one, that is. And it's one page that I've held onto ever since. You see, God did hear my prayers. And although Mom wasn't going home with us, she was certainly going home.

"Our Heavenly Home"

I hear his voice calling me
He's going to take me home
I haven't got a care at all
He's coming very soon
A life of all tranquility
A love that never dies
An everlasting hope for all
Our light will be his eyes
The golden road of life above

Don't Squeeze the Spaceman's Taco

>Keeps going on and on
>A morning star for each new day
>A newness will be born
>The living water overflows
>The road will never end
>Hosanna in the highest place
>His angel he will send
>The strength of all tomorrow too
>There's none that can compare
>I'll see a new horizon soon
>He wants us all to share
>
>*Helen Melerine*

Pookie peers towards me as if focusing on every word that I speak. He then just closes his eyes and smiles. As he does this, a magnificent unrestrained joy lights up the room. Years of worry, heartache and pain – the usual baggage that a parent carries; suddenly all replaced with peace.

I stand there beside Pookie's bed with my hand holding his. It's the same way that I held Mom's hand -- right along the fingertips.

"We're going to be all right." I tell him.

He remains lying with his eyes closed and smiling.

"Well, I know you're not worried about me. But please know that Tyler and Summer are surrounded by people that love them."

His eyes open slightly; just enough to give me a condescending look. "I know." With his opposite hand, he pulls himself towards the handrail. "I just have two things to tell you."

"What's that?" I ask.

"You're wrong and you're right." He leans back and laughs himself into a coughing frenzy.

"I'm scared to ask." I tell him.

Grabbing his bed pan he spits up a bit and clears his throat. There's an orange tinge from the Popsicle that he'd been chewing.

"You're wrong," he tells me. "I do worry about you." Curling his finger, he signals me closer.

I lean in as he looks up towards my forehead.

"And you're right… It does look like a hairy tattoo."

And that was the last Thanksgiving Pookie and I spent together. He passed away shortly after midnight. It was just like him to hold out until after the holiday; to avoid ruining the special day for everyone else. Pookie came into my life in 1985 when he tapped me on my shoulder in algebra class. Lucky for me, algebra just wasn't his thing. Gently, I slid my paper to the side giving him a full view of the correct answers. (A+B= a lifetime of memories). Who says you gain nothing from cheating? I gained a best friend, brother and side kick. Dwayne aka Marcel aka Pookie, I may have helped you get through math class but you helped me get through life. When you feel a tap on your shoulder in that big classroom in the sky, please slide your paper to the side for me. Love you brother. May you forever rest in peace.

The "H" Word Ever After

Epilogue

My heart goes out to the parents of children with severe disabilities. They will never have the peace of knowing that one day their children can survive on their own. My mother had that peace. She may have let her religious expectations beat her down and break her but her faith kept her strong. Her faith let her know that my siblings and I would be all right. Her faith also let her know that she would be all right.

Time passes and I'm determined to live life to the fullest; to never back down and to face the scariest of all challenges head on.

"Brett," I knock on his bedroom door. "Let's go out for a driving lesson."

He may have plowed through a flower bed or two. But then again, they shouldn't have been planted so close to the street.

"You know Kells?" Keeping his eyes on the road Brett continues. "I'm such a good driver and I got such a style."

"Yes you do." I agree while digging my fingernails into the palms of my hands. "Yes you do."

That Christmas I bought Brett the complete *Mario Kart* video game collection. After all, practice makes perfect and future collisions with the neighbor's inflatable Santa Claus should be avoided if at all possible.

Kelly Jude Melerine

Spring arrives and the days become warmer. Birds sing. Flowers bloom. Allergies blossom. Cade has a migraine. And I decide to write about it.

My name is Kelly Jude Melerine and I'm a stay at home dad of a teenage boy with autism named Cade. I quit my job in banking following an extremely rough phase with him. Since then I've become a jack of all trades just to pay the bills. I juggle many tasks so that I may keep a flexible schedule and continue my daily focus on my son. My wife Julee maintains her job as an office manager. Her job provides additional income for the family as well as medical benefits. My son has made tremendous progress with me at home but it's a constant struggle. However, it's a struggle that I will gladly face for him each day.

I decided to set up a blog in hopes of helping others in similar situations. A couple weeks ago I made the first step by establishing the blog. I just haven't been very motivated to write anything since then. Well it is now 1:26 am and Cade has been spitting non-stop for the past hour and a half. In addition to autism Cade suffers from migraines and with his limited verbal abilities he doesn't quite know how to say how badly he feels. I finally got him to take a bath a few minutes ago. A warm bath tends to help comfort him. I'm just waiting for the pain reliever to kick in so that my buddy gets back to his usual giggly self.

Don't Squeeze the Spaceman's Taco

So why the title "Squeeze the Spaceman's Taco?" I am not sure what it means but it's a phrase Cade says and then cracks up laughing. And when Cade cracks up, I crack up. It's really a beautiful thing. There are many other unique phrases of his and I'll tell you about them one day. Life with Cade is anything but boring.

I now hear him saying happy phrases. "Happy," by the way is a word that I'm not allowed to use. I'll tell you about that one day as well. These "H" word phrases of his are signs that the pain has subsided and my giggly buddy is back. There are certain things that Cade says when he's feeling bad and certain things he says when he's feeling good. These phrases may appear to be of little to no significance. However, in my son's world they mean everything. I hope you enjoy this journey into Cade's world. Autism has many sides and I intend to share them all with you; the good and the bad. Now off to get him to bed and hopefully we all get some sleep.

The pollen finally settles and springtime with allergies transitions into summertime with Nana. We load our vehicle and I drive Cade to my sister's house in Middle of Nowhere, Mississippi. Before heading back to our home in North Carolina, I stop to visit my parents. It's a peaceful place, the perfect spot for the two of them. Just a few miles down the road from where we grew up, the family tomb sits among the lush greenery of St. Bernard Catholic Cemetery. They're surrounded by friends and family and right across Bayou Road from St. Bernard Catholic Church.

Mémère Mary used to always ask me, after Mom passed away, if I dreamed of my mother. "Yes," I'd say just to satisfy her. The truth is those dreams were few and far between. My grandmother would then follow by asking me what my mom had to say. I always found that odd – talking to the dead. Yet here I am over twenty years later, and Mom and I talk all the time. I now wonder if Mémère asks Mom the same about me.

You see, Mom's poetry keeps her very much alive. Our late night talks have helped me to get through even the worst of times. I keep a collection of her poetry in the drawer next to my bed. There's comfort in knowing that she'll always be with me. Not just on paper or even handheld electronics thanks to modern technology, but through my many magnificent memories of her.

The leaves change colors making it look as if God sprinkled a box of Fruity Pebbles across His beautiful planet. It's autumn in the Carolinas. Cade is back in school and I'm busy with home repairs and yardwork. Julee picked up some potted mums from the local nursery and I place them along the front sidewalk.

The morning is still young and I go inside for a cup of coffee. It feels good to sit in silence for a moment. My head leans back atop the sofa cushion. Looking out the picture window I watch as the leaves slowly fall. Quickly, Brett comes into view stampeding his usual path down the driveway. His pudgy belly leads the way as he gallops around the sidewalk's edge.

"Listen Kells," he tells me while opening the front door. "About those new plants… I didn't do it."

Thanksgiving rolls back around and only two mums have survived. Our home is filled with the things that make the holiday special.

- Family

- Turkey
- Some gravy for Brett
- A mixture of Lebanese and Creole dishes
- And of course the stories -- the many splendid stories that keep the family alive.

They live. Mom lives on through the art of her poetic words. Julee's mother lives through the recipes on the table set before us. Her father and mine both live through the laughs that we share when we talk about their flaring tempers.

"You sound just like your dad," is all that it takes for us both to simmer down.

They live. They live through the most unexpected little things that remind us of them

My brother Larry was my most recent loved one to pass. What was it like having a brother 14 years older?

> Larry: Hey Kelly you want to make $5.
> Me: Sure.
> Larry: Smell my feet and tell me which one smells worse. If you pick the right one, you get $5.
> Me: Bring on those feet!

That left foot smelled like a cross between 8 day old road kill and moldy goat cheese. The right foot, although rancid, was not quite as bad.

> Me: (With a bit of vomit in my mouth.) The left one is definitely worse.
> Larry: No you didn't pick the right foot so you lose.

I can't tell you how many times I lost out on that money making opportunity. No matter how often Larry conned me, I fell for it every time. It's funny the things we miss in this crazy life. Larry was the type of person that would make Jerry Springer blush. He was a great role model for me growing up (of what not to do). All I can say is that I love him and my heart is crushed. But I know that one day I will smell those disgusting putrid feet once more. And Larry, if you're listening, you better pay up.

They live. They live through the hearts of the children that they leave behind.

They live. They live through the extra dinner plates that are no longer needed. One for Pookie and one for Aunt Delores. She's recently passed as well. And although they're no longer physically with us, we've continued to save their places right next to each other at the family table. Well… because we all know the way that Aunt Delores felt about Pookie.

And as for Cade, what lies next for him? Why is there no clear resolution for the main character of whom I write? This is the missing puzzle piece for 1 in 59.

References

- *Aladdin*, Directed by: Ron Clements and John Musker, Written by: Ron Clements, John Musker, Ted Elliott and Terry Rossio, Produced by: Ron Clements and John Musker, Production Company: Walt Disney Pictures and Walt Disney Feature Animation, Distributed by: Buena Vista Pictures, 1992.

- Centers for Disease Control and Prevention, http://www.cdc.gov/ncbddd/autism/data.html , Accessed August 19, 2018.

- "Hakuna Matata," Produced by: Jay Rifkin, Fabian Cooke and Mark Mancina, Written by: Elton John and Tim Rice, From the movie *The Lion King*, Walt Disney Pictures and Walt Disney Feature Animation, 1994.

- *X-Men – The Last Stand*, Directed by: Brett Ratner, Written by: Simon Kinberg and Zak Penn, Produced by: Lauren Shuler Donner, Ralph Winter and Avi Arad, Production Company: Marvel Entertainment, The Donners' Company and Ingenious Film Partners, Distributed by: 20th Century Fox, 2005.

- *Snakes on a Plane*, Directed by: David R. Ellis, Screenplay Written by: David J. Taylor, John Heffernan and Sebastian Gutierrez, Story Written by: David J. Taylor, John Heffernan and David Dalessandro, Produced by: Craig Berenson, Don Granger and Gary Levinson, Production Company: Mutual Film Company, Distributed by: New Line Cinema, 2006.

- *The Little Mermaid*, Directed by: Ron Clements and John Musker, Screenplay written by: Ron Clements and John Musker, Fairy Tale written by: Hans Christian Andersen,

Additional Dialogue by: Howard Ashman, Gerrit Graham, Samuel Graham and Chris Hubbell, Distributed by: Buena Vista Pictures, 1989.

- *Austin Powers - International Man of Mystery*, Directed by: Jay Roach, Written by: Mike Myers, Produced by: Jay Blenkin, Eric McLeod, Demi Moore, Mike Myers, Claire Rudnik Polstein, Production Company: Capella International / KC Medien, Moving Pictures / Eric's Boy, Distributed by: New Line Cinema, 1997.

- *Shrek,* Directed by: Andrew Adamson and Vicky Jenson, Produced by: Jeffrey Katzenberg, Screenplay by: Ted Elliott, Terry Rossio, Joe Stillman and Roger S. H. Schulman, Distributed by: DreamWorks Pictures, 2001.

- *The Dark Knight*, Directed by: Christopher Nolan, Produced by: Emma Thomas, Charles Roven and Christopher Nolan, Screenplay by: Jonathan Nolan and Christopher Nolan, Distributed by: Warner Brothers Pictures, 2008.

- "I GARONTEE," Justin Wilson - Cajun chef and humorist, Born April 24, 1914 – Died September 5, 2001, http://justinwilson.com

- *Toy Story,* Directed by: John Lasseter, Produced by: Ralph Guggenheim and Bonnie Arnold, Screenplay by: Joss Whedon, Andrew Stanton, Joel Cohen and Alec Sokolow, Distributed by: Buena Vista Pictures, 1995.

- *The Nightmare Before Christmas,* Directed by: Henry Selick, Produced by: Tim Burton and Denise Di Novi, Screenplay by: Caroline Thompson, Story by: Michael McDowell Distributed by: Buena Vista Pictures, 1993.

- *Driving Miss Daisy,* Directed by: Bruce Beresford, Produced by: Richard D Zanuck and Lili Fini Zanuck, Screenplay by: Alfred Unry, Distributed by: Warner Bros, 1989.

- *"I spontaneously bust out in Ninja moves"* is a quote found on packets of Border Sauce. Border Sauce is a product of Taco Bell – a subsidiary of Yum! Headquartered in Irvine, CA, Founded in 1962.

- *Rocky,* Directed by: John G. Avildsen, Produced by: Robert Chartoff and Irwin Winkler, Written by: Sylvester Stallone, Distributed by: United Artists, 1976.

- "E.T.," Produced by: Dr. Luke, Ammo and Max Martin, Written by: Katy Perry, Lukasz Gottwald, Max Martin, Joshua Coleman and Kanye West, From the album *Teenage Dream*, Label: Capitol Records, 2010.

- *"Roaches check in, but they don't check out!,"* is a product slogan for the Roach Motel brand of insect traps trademarked in May 1976 by Black Flag insecticide brand. Black Flag was acquired by Spectrum Brands in 2011.

- *"The best a man can get,"* is a product slogan for the Gilette brand of men's razors which was launched during the Super Bowl of 1989. Gilette was owned by The Gilette Company which was later acquired by Proctor & Gamble in 2005.

Made in the USA
Middletown, DE
30 April 2019